C000152111

The Dark Side
Part 2

**Real Life Accounts of an NHS Paramedic
The Traumatic, the Tragic and the Tearful**

by bestselling British author

Andy Thompson

****

Also Available

The Dark Side

Real Life Accounts of an NHS Paramedic

The Good, the Bad and the Downright Ugly

Published in September 2014 by emp3books,
Norwood House, Elvetham Road, Fleet, GU51 4HL, England

The Dark Side Part 2

Real Life Accounts of an NHS Paramedic
The Traumatic, the Tragic and the Tearful
by Andy Thompson

Copyright © Andy Thompson 2014 - All rights reserved.
Digital edition first published in 2014 by The Electronic Book
Company

ISBN: 978-1-907140-46-4

Dedication

This book is dedicated to my beautiful wife, Emma, for her encouragement and support throughout its production; and to all those Health Care Professionals around the globe who, where possible, save life and work tirelessly to help make a difference to their sick and injured patients.

About the Author

In June 2002, Andy commenced employment with the Mersey Regional Ambulance Service, which later merged with the Cumbria, Greater Manchester and Lancashire Ambulance Services to form the Northwest Ambulance Service NHS Trust. He rapidly progressed from the Patient Transport Service (PTS) to qualified Paramedic status via Ambulance Technician training, experience gained in the job and further extended training from which, upon qualifying, he was presented with a 'Professional Paramedic Development Award' for most improved candidate.

In 2005 he registered with the Health Professions Council (HPC), the national governing body for UK paramedics; this changed its name to the Health and Care Professions Council (HCPC) in August 2012.

Andy spent the earlier part of his career working in the English counties of Cheshire and Merseyside. In 2007, after living 'up north' for 32 years, Andy relocated down south with his wife and two children, residing there until he and his family relocated to North Yorkshire in September 2013. There, Andy continues his career as an NHS Paramedic with the Yorkshire Ambulance Service.

To read more about the author, please visit:
www.andythompson-author.com

Contents

The Dark Side

Prologue

The incidents I have written about in this book are a selection of real life accounts of situations I have experienced during my career in the NHS Ambulance Service. And although they are not all necessarily adrenal-fuelled encounters, they're still experiences that have remained with me through no choice of my own; they've become engraved for one reason only – because they are all unforgettable. Therefore, what is written is as true and honest as my long-term memory allows. And with the exception of chapter 3, the accounts told are supported by the *precise* details taken from anonymised copies of the official NHS documentation I recorded at the time of each incident. Furthermore, the dialogue quoted in each chapter is also true to what remains in my long-term memory; however, I do not profess it to be verbatim.

The Dark Side

.

Introduction

'The Dark Side' – an unofficial term used by Mersey Regional Ambulance Service personnel to describe the career transition from the non-emergency aspect, to the frontline emergency aspect, of the Ambulance Service; pertaining to the fact that what one frequently encounters is often a grim and sombre experience.

Paramedics often refer to themselves as a *'Jack of All Trades, Master of None'*. Speaking as a professionally registered paramedic myself, that statement couldn't be closer to the truth. One minute you're dispatched to a patient with chest pain, potentially suffering from a heart attack, and you assume the role of an unqualified Cardiologist. An hour or so later you're dispatched to an imminent birth and you adopt the role of an unqualified Midwife. One cup of tea later, if you're lucky, you're hurtling towards the address of a patient who wants to end their life, and so you play the role of an unqualified Counsellor. You then neck a bit of scran, if you're very lucky, and soon find yourself compressing the chest of an elderly patient in cardiac arrest, and so don the cap of a Resuscitation Officer for an hour. Furthermore, with the amount of drugs we now carry, paramedics frequently administer controlled medicines, and therefore play the role of an unqualified Dispensing Pharmacist too. I could go on and on but I'm sure you get my point.

Even if paramedics are a 'Jack of All Trades, Master of None', the Ambulance Service is, strictly speaking, classed as an 'Essential Service', as opposed to what it is more commonly known as, an Emergency Service – though I would say all of the emergency services are 'essential'. Without the Ambulance Service, hundreds of thousands of people would die unnecessarily every year, and so, on a global scale, the Service makes a significant difference to people's lives every day of the year.

However, with all that said, I'm often told by friends, family and, bizarrely enough, by some of my patients, that my job is a thankless one. I'm not asked if *I* think it is, I'm simply told it is. Nevertheless, I feel compelled to disagree with them all. I can't speak for all ambulance personnel but I cannot possibly even estimate the number of times that I've been thanked personally by patients or their loved ones. OK, we may not get as many 'Thank You' letters as ward nurses do but that's understandable, because patients are only in our care for an hour or so, whereas nurses often care for patients for weeks or even months at a time.

Even if my job was a thankless one, I wouldn't want to work in any other profession at this current time in my working life. That said, I've come very close to having to. Why? Because there have been moments throughout my career when I've sat on the back step of an ambulance parked outside of an A&E department, with my head in my hands and a bucket full of adrenaline still hurtling through my veins, and thought, 'I'm not sure if I can do this anymore'. Fortunately though, those thoughts usually only arose after I'd been party to an extremely sombre incident, particularly where a child was involved, and it would pass after I helped bring another new life into the world, reduced somebody's unbearable pain, saved a life, consoled a deceased patient's loved one, or gave a live-alone, frail OAP a little TLC. Or simply made the difference to a suicidal youth's state of mind – often just a listening ear or a little life-advice is all that is needed there.

So, not having deviated just yet from what is becoming an ever-increasingly demanding profession, mentally and physically, I'm very pleased to share with you another selection of *'Real Life Accounts'*. And in this second instalment, there's once again Trauma, Tragedy and Tears.

Delivered in a style similar to my first book, I hope to provide another thought provoking and thorough insight into the harrowing experiences that paramedics have to frequently endure, and I explain each incident informatively and in graphic detail, while of course keeping the lay person reader in mind.

No heroics were performed during the incidents recounted in this book; I simply did my job and what is expected of me during each shift. I did and thought – clinically, that is – what *most* paramedics around the globe would do and think, and I'm sure *most* paramedics will relate to the incidents contained within.

So, are you ready? Come on, don that fluorescent jacket for a second time – you know, the one with 'Observer' emblazoned across the back – grab yourself a cuppa, sit back, put your feet up and imagine you're on duty with me, experiencing another selection of my Real Life Accounts.

The Dark Side

Chapter 1
Blackout

We're very fortunate in the UK that the NHS operates twenty-four-seven, three hundred and sixty-five days of the year. Granted, summer is the best part of the year for paramedics because we occasionally get to relax in the sun and sit on standby, 'people watching', while eating an ice-cream; fantastic! Though, I've had to dispose of a lot of ice-creams prematurely in order to promptly respond to an emergency call. Spring and autumn are not too bad either, but winter, however, can be hell! It's freezing cold on a day shift, even colder on a night shift, and when it snows, good grief! Mother Nature cuts the emergency services no slack whatsoever.

Regardless of poor weather conditions, people obviously get sick and have accidents and subsequently ring treble-nine. Winter weather can sometimes make the job of ambulance crews very difficult. There are increased risks associated with driving, and with access and egress to and from patients' homes, particularly egressing, as carrying patients in the carry-chair down snow covered or frozen-over concrete steps, driveways and pavements, etcetera, is often very daunting. I've known many accidents to happen, some of which resulted in ambulance personnel getting injured badly enough to have no choice but to go on long-term sickness leave. Nevertheless, it's a risk that ambulance personnel have to take to help patients who need us at their worst hour, as the following patient did in the early hours of a cold winter morning while I was on a night shift.

It was 2:40 a.m. and it had been snowing for most of the night, and it still was. There was a good few inches of snow spread like a blanket all over the grounds of the ambulance station and beyond. I was on station in the mess room, power-napping, sat with three of my colleagues, including fellow paramedic and my crewmate, Adele. The night had been quite busy thus far and I was beginning to wilt a bit through sheer exhaustion. My brain did not feel ready to be taxed for the remainder of the shift. I began feeling a little restless and therefore decided to go outside for some fresh air and to admire the crisp, white snow. Actually, as I've mentioned snow, I'll have to tell you a little humorous anecdote a former colleague told me when I was working as a postman. It went something like this.

Before my friend was a postman, he worked for a well-known brewery. Upon him finishing a night shift at seven o'clock in the morning, he clocked-off along with his work mates and exited the premises, and although he knew it had been snowing, he was surprised to see it had snowed as much as it had, so much in fact that he was able to make decent sized snowballs. While several of his colleagues had an early morning snowball fight, he walked towards his car parked on the roadside, talking to a female colleague as he strolled along, casually picking up snow as they conversed. When he arrived at his car he said goodbye and parted from her.

She continued to amble towards her car a short distance away. As she got into her car, her back to my friend, he threw a snowball in her direction. Proceeding to slam the car door shut, some snow went into the foot-well. Not knowing who had thrown it, and without observing for any passing vehicles, she abruptly opened the door to remove the snow from inside her car. At the same time, another car drove past on her side of the road. BANG! The passing car took her door clean off its hinges.

Having heard the bang and the shocked woman's scream, her colleagues, including my friend, went over to help and calm her. However, to the present day he has never told her that it was him who threw the snowball. I absolutely love it when would-be harmless pranks go wrong; it makes them all the funnier.

Anyway, after standing outside for ten minutes watching the snow fall heavily, and having inhaled some fresh air, I went back into the mess room and offered to make tea. I often make tea while on station just for the sake of it, because you never know when, or even where your next cup is coming from. I do occasionally accept the offer of a brew in a patient's house, but only if I can assess and treat them at home... and as long as they're not mingers!

I entered the kitchen. If it had been a very busy previous seventy-two hours or so for the crews, it sometimes resembled the kitchen from the politically incorrect, yet hilarious UK sitcom *The Young Ones.* So I began the challenge of looking for clean cups that didn't have deep tannin stains embedded, or Penicillin growing inside them. I'm serious! I don't know if it's just the ambulance service or all of the emergency services, but trying to find clean crockery in the station kitchen is like looking for a virgin in a maternity ward.

So, stood alone in the kitchen, I ascertained my fellow colleagues' tea preferences. And as per usual, ascertaining tea preferences from the crew I was working with that particular night would have gone something like this:

'How do you want yours, Bill?' I'd shout through to the mess room.

'Julie Andrews for me please, Andy,' he'd say, meaning 'white nun'. 'Don't make it fortnight tea though, will you.' By that he meant not too weak.

'OK, how about you, Adele?' I'd ask.

'Arnie please,' she'd say, meaning she wanted hers strong. Who would think you could speak in code making a simple cup of tea, hey!

I didn't get a chance to make a brew because Adele and I were dispatched to a fifty-seven year old male complaining of chest pain, before I'd even had the chance to finish washing the cups to an acceptable state to drink from. We promptly vacated the station and Adele drove towards the address given to us, using blue lights, but she refrained from using the sirens. Due to the poor weather conditions, Adele had little choice but to drive slowly, and to gently navigate around bends and use deceleration to slow down, as opposed to frequent use of the brakes, to minimise the risk of skidding.

When we arrived at the address, we grabbed the bare essential equipment only, not because we were being lazy but because chest pain is better assessed and treated in the ambulance; we therefore intended to get the patient into the ambulance as soon as possible. Between us both, we carried the Entonox – a.k.a 'gas and air' – a carry-chair, two blankets and the ECG machine and walked towards the house along the snow covered driveway.

The ECG machine can not only be used to analyse a patient's heart rhythm, but can be used to 'shock' – or defibrillate, to be precise – a patient who goes in to cardiac arrest, providing that they present in one of two arrhythmias where defibrillation is an appropriate form of medical intervention; that is Ventricular

Fibrillation (VF) or *Pulseless* Ventricular Tachycardia (VT). I say *pulseless* because a person can present with VT but have a pulse and be fully conscious, and therefore does not meet the criteria for defibrillation.

When we arrived at the front door, we were welcomed by a lady, the patient's wife. She escorted us to the large lounge where the patient, George, was sat down on the sofa, dressed in his PJ's. I took one look at him and thought, 'Heart Attack!' Amongst other tell-tale signs, he was holding his clenched fist close to his chest. That single gesture of body language put my diagnostic senses on heightened alert, because that is a typical sign of someone experiencing crushing-like chest pain.

Chest pain is a cardinal sign of a heart attack, or myocardial infarction (MI), to be precise. However, chest pain can also be the sign of numerous other conditions, some life-threatening and others not so life-threatening. Nevertheless, when someone rings treble-nine and mentions chest pain, the caller is questioned from the highest acuity to the lowest acuity, but in most cases an ambulance is dispatched immediately – regardless of the patient's age – just in case it is a heart attack that is causing the patient's chest pain.

Looking directly at George, I immediately noticed his face was ashen and he was sweating profusely. His facial expression was that of someone frightened to death... no, frightened *of* death would be a better description. That is known in medical textbooks as 'a fear of impending doom', and it's a very unpleasant sight to witness, let alone be the person actually feeling it. His breathing was quite shallow, partly due to anxiety, but perhaps more so due to his struggling heart trying to provide enough oxygenated blood to the vital organs of his body. Adele and I looked at each other, instantly acknowledging George's death-like appearance. His presentation caused me to get ahead of myself a little and I started to think about all the basic and advanced skills and observations that we were going to have to do, on top of a myriad of drugs we would need to administer if my suspicions were correct. And they would need undertaking fast. 'I want him in the ambulance A-S-A-P!' I thought.

I sat down on the sofa next to George and applied a pair of disposable, protective nitrile gloves. Remaining calm, with Adele and George's wife stood beside me, I introduced myself and Adele. Then, using implied consent, I took hold of his wrist to feel for an approximate rate and strength of his pulse. While doing that, I could feel he was very sweaty and clammy to the touch; in fact, that's an understatement, he was wringing wet through, his pyjama top was clinging to his body like Lycra. With his initial presentation mentally noted, I then began to ascertain some pertinent history from him, with regards to the background events that had resulted in a treble-nine call being made.

'George, you're holding your chest, I take it you still have chest pain, is that right?' I asked, knowing full well what his answer would be, but didn't want to assume.

'Yeah,' he replied, with a look of fear on his face and sweat dripping down his pale forehead.

As George still had pain, I immediately asked Adele to get me a *sats*, also known as *SP02*, which is placed on a digit, usually the index finger, to measure how well the blood circulating around the body is being oxygenated. It also attempts to display a pulse rate, although the pulse measurement is rarely accurate. Normal saturations of oxygen would be between ninety-five and one hundred percent on atmospheric air. While Adele waited for George's sats to display, I asked her to prepare and hand over the Entonox to him to self-administer of his own free will. Entonox is an analgesic usually offered to women in labour, but is also frequently used as an initial pain relief for chest pain, or other pain such as limb fractures, until IV access is obtained. Then, if appropriate, a more potent intravenous analgesic can be administered in addition to Entonox.

George began self-administering the Entonox while I continued to palpate the rate and strength of his pulse. It felt slow and weak. That concerned me a lot and caused me to consider deviating slightly from the normal procedure undertaken for a patient with chest pain, particularly a heart attack; that is, until I could confirm whether my suspicions were correct or not. I pondered for a moment, 'What if George is having a heart attack, where is the occlusion? His pulse is slow and weak. What if it is in the inferior (lower) part of his heart; that would mean certain drugs might make his condition even worse.' What I needed was a blood pressure and an ECG to enable me to select and administer the right treatment to George. Directing my gaze at Adele, I asked,

'Can you take his blood pressure, hun?' Then I glanced back at George and asked, 'What time did the pain come on, George?' Momentarily releasing his lips from the Entonox mouthpiece, he answered,

'About an hour ago, it woke me up.'

'OK, does anything improve the pain, like leaning forward?' I asked. George leant forward,

'No,' he said, before inhaling on the Entonox again.

'Does anything make the pain worse, like taking a deep breath in?' He took an exaggerated deep breath, which is what I wanted him to do.

'No,' he answered.

'How would you describe the pain: dull, tight, crushing?' I asked with relevance.

'Crushing, like someone is hugging me too hard.'

'And does the pain radiate anywhere?'

'Down my arm and in my jaw,' he answered, rubbing the palm of his right hand down his left arm.

Pain down the arm, particularly the left arm, and in the jaw is a common complaint from a patient suffering from a heart attack; although that can also be a typical complaint of a cardiac condition called angina. That is where the blood flow to the heart via a coronary artery is partially restricted, as opposed to being completely restricted, as in a *typical* heart attack. Angina can be a pre-cursor to a full-blown heart attack, particularly if the angina-like pain comes on at rest. However, if angina pain comes on during mild exertion, it is commonly treated by the patient with a drug called Glycerol Tri-nitrate, or GTN for short. GTN is a potent vasodilator, which means when sprayed under the patient's tongue it causes arteries to dilate, thus allowing an adequate amount of oxygenated blood to flow to the heart.

Due to George complaining of pain in the jaw and down his arm, and that it had come on at rest, I was becoming more and more convinced that he was having a heart attack and so proceeded to treat him for one. Still sat beside him on the sofa, I continued to question him further.

'George, can you take aspirin, you're not allergic to it are you? Or do you have any active gastric ulcers, or are you on any blood thinners such as warfarin?'

'No, I can take aspirin,' he answered in a breathless manner. So I removed an aspirin from its packaging and handed it to George to chew, then progressed with my initial assessment and treatment for a suspected, but as yet unconfirmed, heart attack.

'Now, on a scale of zero to ten, ten being the worst pain you have ever been in, how would you score the crushing chest pain that you have right now?'

'Ten,' he said with clear certainty.

'Do you feel nauseas at all, or have you vomited since the pain came on?'

'No,' he said, shaking his head, still with the 'fear of impending doom' expression on his face.

Following that questioning, my suspicions had risen even further. Based on his ashen and sweaty appearance and his answers, I was pretty confident that George was having a heart attack. If my suspicions were correct, he could deteriorate to a cardiac arrest within minutes and I didn't want that happening while we were in the house. Actually, I didn't want that to happen at all! But if it did, as previously mentioned, carrying patients in the carry-chair down snow covered or frozen-over concrete steps is often very daunting, but carrying a 'dead weight' from the house in the snow and ice is fraught with danger and a whole lot more difficult than with a 'live' patient. Plus, because the ground was layered with snow, it would make wheeling the carry-chair across the driveway to the ambulance a lot more difficult too.

George was a time-critical patient and needed to receive the appropriate pre-hospital treatment and conveying to hospital fast!

'Right, do you have any other medical conditions at all, George?'

'He's diabetic,' his wife answered before George even had chance to.

'Do you take insulin, George?'

'Yeah… It's in the fridge if you need it,' his wife answered again, as if performing a ventriloquist act with her husband.

'No, that's fine,' I said to her, before directing my eyes at Adele,

'What's his blood pressure, hun?'

'One hundred over sixty, and his sats are ninety-six percent on gas 'n' air. The sats monitor is showing a pulse rate of fifty,' she replied.

'Cheers, hun. His pulse felt slower than that to me though,' I replied.

A normal adult 'textbook' systolic blood pressure would be one hundred and twenty millimetres of mercury, or 120mmHg. A systolic below 90mmHg is considered low blood pressure, particularly if symptoms are present. Systolic means the arterial pressure during contraction of the heart. It is measured in 'millimetres of mercury', pertaining to the fact that sphygmomanometers – the equipment used for measuring blood pressure – historically contained mercury, hence the letters 'mmHg' following the preceding figure.

George's sats were a little low at ninety-six percent, considering he was inhaling Entonox, which contains oxygen. However, I wasn't overly concerned by that measurement. My main concern was George's blood pressure, as it was quite low for his age. Normally, paramedics would administer a dose of GTN to a patient with chest pain of cardiac origin, because, as already mentioned, GTN is a vasodilator which dilates the arteries; that alone can reduce chest pain as more oxygenated blood can reach the tissues of the heart, feeding it with the nutrients it needs to sustain its pumping action. But to safely administer GTN, your patient's systolic blood pressure must be above ninety, because the dilating effects of GTN can cause blood pressure to reduce significantly. George's systolic blood pressure was 100mmHg, but while that was OK, I was concerned about the correlation of his low blood pressure and slow heart rate. Administering GTN to a patient with a slow heart rate and low blood pressure could cause him to 'crash', for want of a better word. I had to consider my next step promptly but carefully.

Adele, having heard George's wife say that her husband was diabetic, gained consent and pin-pricked his finger for a drop of blood to measure his blood glucose. She then informed me that the glucometer displayed a figure of 22 millimoles per litre of blood, which is usually written as mmol/l. That was high and spoke volumes to my provisional diagnosis. You see, the cause of high blood sugar levels in a diabetic can be due to a heart attack, often a 'silent' heart attack. By silent I mean the patient does not feel chest pain. It is common for diabetics to suffer a heart attack either with or without chest pain – without chest pain due to neuropathy. Neuropathy causes impairment or even absence of various sensations, one of them being pain, so the nerves do not transmit pain sensation to the brain to be interpreted. In other cases, diabetics feel chest pain but with the absence of one or more of the other textbook signs and symptoms of a heart attack. For example: pale, sweaty and clammy skin; nausea, vomiting, double incontinence; and fear of impending doom. George did present with fear of impending doom, and was pale, sweaty and had clammy skin, but he didn't complain of nausea. And fortunately for him, Adele and me, he hadn't vomited or been incontinent of urine or faeces.

We had been on scene with George for just several minutes. Adele had already pre-empted the removal of George by carry-chair and had therefore prepared it. George may have been completely independent and able to mobilise, but allowing him to walk to the ambulance could have caused him to exert himself, which would have placed more strain on his already struggling heart, so the use of the carry-chair was an absolute necessity. George came to his feet and then sat himself on the carry-chair, still holding his fist across his chest. I wrapped him in a blanket, placed the safety strap across him and fastened it, but left his right hand free so he could continue inhaling the Entonox as he felt the need. Carefully but quickly, I wheeled him from the lounge, down the hallway, towards the front door. Adele and I then lifted the carry-chair, with George in situ, up and over the threshold and down the snow covered concrete steps. The snow was still falling heavily, so with my head down and eyes squinting I pulled the chair backwards, as opposed to the usual method of pushing the chair forward, along the driveway towards the ambulance. His concerned wife locked the front door and followed closely behind, kindly carrying some of our equipment.

For the short scurry to the ambulance, I kept a close watch on George's conscious level as best as I could, as it was dark and the street lighting was quite poor. When we reached the ambulance, Adele opened the rear saloon doors and lowered the ramp. I then pulled the chair in a reverse manner into the artificially lit saloon of the ambulance.

'OK George, can you pop yourself onto the stretcher, please,' I said, unclipping the safety straps from around him. George came to his feet and lay semi-recumbent on the stretcher, while Adele raised the ramp and shut the rear doors. George's wife, looking very troubled, sat down and kept very quiet so Adele and I could continue with our assessment and treatment. Time was of the essence and George needed to be conveyed to hospital with as little delay as possible. But before we could begin mobilising to hospital, we needed to undertake further observations on him, as one particular test required the vehicle to be stationary for it to measure accurately, and also for it to print legibly. That was a 12-Lead ECG.

A 12-Lead ECG only has 10 leads but it analyses the rhythm of the heart from 12 different angles. It is used to assist a paramedic, and various other health care professionals, to diagnose a number of cardiac conditions. However, its primary purpose is to diagnose a heart attack. So, undertaking an ECG would, in *most* cases, enable me to confirm whether George was having a heart attack or not. It would also enable me to analyse his exact heart rate, which I was certain was very slow. In addition to a 12-Lead ECG, we also had to administer further drugs, including another analgesic, as Entonox was not providing adequate pain relief for him.

With Adele by my side, I asked her to obtain IV access, which involves inserting a needle into a vein, then withdrawing the needle, leaving a clear plastic tube in place through which drugs and/or fluids can be administered. Meanwhile, I wrapped the automatic blood pressure cuff, which comes attached to the ECG monitor, around George's right arm, switched the machine on and pressed the start button. While the blood pressure cuff inflated and tightened around George's arm, I wired him up to the 12-Lead ECG monitor. Moments later, a blood pressure reading appeared on the monitor; by now his systolic measured just 80mmHg.

With that measurement noted, I then observed his heart rate on the screen. To no surprise, my suspicions were confirmed; George's heart rate was just 33 beats per minute (BPM). The monitor was only capable of showing one lead at a time, lead two by default. Nevertheless, upon pressing the 'analyse twelve lead ECG' button it would, in effect, take a 'picture' of the heart from twelve different angles, and I would be able to scrutinise each of twelve different views of the heart individually.

Adele had put a cannula into George's arm, so a patent drug route was available. If my provisional diagnosis turned out to be a definitive diagnosis, he was going to need it. With his consent, I would be administering that many drugs to him in order to save his life that, were they in tablet form, he would rattle like a tube of Smarties when he moved!

'George, I need you to keep still for me now while the ECG analyses your heart, OK? Adele, can you prepare the atropine, metoclopramide and morphine for me as quickly as you can,' I asked by way of an instruction. George took several inhalations of Entonox and then kept still. I pressed the 'analyse twelve lead' button on the monitor and waited for it to print out. Seconds later, the paper began to appear with the results. I tore the long paper strip from the monitor and opened it out in its entirety. What was displayed was no surprise to me whatsoever. I handed the strip to Adele. She glanced down at it and then looked back up at me,

'You'd better get the checklist out, mate,' Adele said, as she stood preparing the drugs I'd requested.

Before I informed George that I had good reason to suspect that he was having a heart attack, and with his wife sat down behind me oblivious to my intentions, I went through a twenty-point checklist of questions to ensure that George met the criteria for thrombolysis. Thrombolysis is a pharmacological procedure which involves administering, via an intravenous route, a drug that costs between £350 and £600 a shot. Tenecteplase – more commonly known to health care professionals as TNK – is a clot-busting drug. If successful, it literally dissolves the clot in the recipient's coronary artery.

Today, most patients will not receive pre-hospital thrombolysis but instead be conveyed by ambulance, under emergency driving conditions, to a catheter laboratory. There they will have an invasive procedure called Primary Percutaneous Coronary Intervention (PPCI). That involves reopening the blocked coronary artery with a 'balloon' and placing one or more stents in the culprit artery. This restores blood supply to the part of the heart that is starved of oxygenated blood. I've watched the procedure being carried out, it's intriguing and the surgeons are without a doubt very clever people indeed.

Following nineteen of twenty positive ticks on the checklist, it was *almost* confirmed that George met the criteria to receive TNK from me, as long as I administered a drug that has a pharmacological purpose of increasing the heart rate and blood pressure. That drug was atropine. Atropine is derived from the plant, *Deadly Nightshade*. It gets its title from the 'correct' name for Deadly Nightshade – *Atropa belladonna*. If I administered atropine to George, it would have to have the desired effect on him in order for me to administer TNK through his veins.

I broke the news to George that I strongly suspected that he was having a heart attack, and that I would like to administer a drug which can destroy the clot that was occluding an artery in his heart. I also had to inform George that a potential side effect of the drug could cause a stroke, which may or may not kill him. Conversely, I also had to explain to him that if he withheld consent for me to thrombolyse him, then the heart attack *could* kill him anyway. That explanation wasn't me being unsympathetic or blunt, it was procedure and his basic human right. A patient has the right to know what the risks are of consenting to such treatment, and the risks associated with refusing treatment too.

George consented, but first I had to administer some atropine through the cannula, so Adele passed me the pre-filled syringe of atropine. I opened up the injection port of the cannula and squeezed 500 micrograms of atropine through his veins, watching the monitor closely for an increase in heart rate, as the drug often takes effect quickly. Administering atropine to your patient is, in effect, like injecting poison into them; it feels quite eerie really, poisoning a patient in order to save their life, but that's what's fascinating about medicine. What would we do without pharmacists and researchers, hey? They're absolutely brilliant!

With my eyes fixed on the monitor, George's heart rate gradually increased to 57 BPM. 'Brilliant,' I thought. I measured George's blood pressure for a third time. That too had increased, to 110mmHg. Adele then passed me the drugs that she had prepared for me moments earlier; they were metoclopramide – an anti-sickness/nausea drug – and morphine. My intention was to reduce George's pain score to a zero, if possible, before I pushed the TNK drug through the cannula in his arm. So I initially administered 10 milligrams of metoclopramide over two minutes, followed by an initial 2.5 milligrams dose of morphine. Laying semi-recumbent on the stretcher, George informed me that he could no longer tolerate inhaling Entonox, therefore I replaced the oxygen he was getting from the Entonox with supplemental oxygen via a face mask.

Thus far, he had received Entonox, oxygen, aspirin, atropine, metoclopramide and morphine. His pain score had only reduced to a five out of ten following the initial dose of the opiate-based analgesic. I pondered for a moment, 'Should I give him some GTN? Doing so would act as another analgesic, as more oxygenated blood would reach his struggling heart, but it may also lower his blood pressure again due to its effect on the arteries. Then again, if it did, I could add a little more atropine to the cocktail of drugs I'd already administered.' So I momentarily removed the O2 mask from George's face and sprayed a dose of GTN under his tongue, followed by a further 2.5 milligrams of IV morphine. Administering that second dose required me to closely monitor his respiratory rate and sats.

Adele, knowing full well that George had met the criteria to receive the TNK, had prepared the appropriate dose for his estimated weight, and also the correct dose of the drug heparin. Heparin is a blood thinning drug, similar to warfarin, and is used alongside TNK. Prior to administering TNK, heparin is given via the IV route.

I held the heparin syringe in my right hand and glanced at George again; he was still sweaty and clammy but appeared better than he had when we first arrived at his side. His improved appearance was due to the morphine, Entonox, oxygen and an increased heart rate and blood pressure from the effects of atropine. I glanced at the ECG print-out laid flat on the work surface in the saloon of the ambulance. Despite the fact that Adele, also a paramedic, believed George was having a heart attack, for a moment I doubted both hers and my own diagnosis. I glanced at the ECG once again to reaffirm to myself that it definitely displayed the signs of a massive heart attack. 'Yes, I'm sure of it,' I thought, as last second nerves tried to get the better of me.

It's not as if it was the first time I'd diagnosed a heart attack or treated a patient with TNK, but it was nerve-wracking every time the predicament arose. The patient's life is not only in your hands but heavily reliant on your level of understanding of patient presentations, signs, symptoms, and your skill, knowledge and ability to interpret the ECG. It's also an unpleasant feeling knowing that once the drug is pushed through the patient's veins, you can't take it back out. If my diagnosis was wrong and George's ashen, sweaty and clammy appearance was due to another cause, and what appeared on his ECG print-out was actually caused by another condition commonly known as an MI imposter, then pushing the drug through could potentially cost George his life. But every second that went by meant a part of George's heart was being starved of oxygen, so I just had to trust my knowledge and skills, go with my gut instinct, and just do it. After all, there is a saying in the medical profession, *'if it looks like a duck, quacks like a duck and tastes good with orange sauce, then it's a duck'.*

With that saying flooding my mind, I flicked open the cap of the cannula and held the syringe in my right hand, then positioned it vertically into the injection port. 'Here we go,' I thought. As I squeezed the pump of the syringe, well aware that my hands were shaking and my heart rate had increased with the circumstantial adrenaline flow, I watched the contents of heparin empty into George's veins. Then, I flushed the drug through with a little sodium chloride. Adele then passed me the syringe containing the TNK. With my hands still shaking a little, I immediately squeezed the TNK through the cannula, once again followed by a small amount of flush. The contents were gone. There was no going back now, and no way to remove the clot-busting drug from George's circulatory system.

'That's it, George,' I said, alternating my gaze between him and his wife, 'the clot-busting drug is in your veins, so relax as best you can and let it do its job.'

We'd been treating George in the back of the ambulance for fifteen minutes when Adele peered outside through the saloon window.

'Bloody 'ell, we'd better get moving, Andy,' she said, with a look of concern on her face because of how much snow had fallen since we had mobilised from the ambulance station.

'OK, you jump up front then and alert the CCU for me, will you. I'll give you a shout when I'm ready to move off,' I said. By CCU I meant the Cardiac Care Unit. At the time, that was the normal place to convey a patient who had been diagnosed in a pre-hospital environment as having a heart attack, and had received TNK. Adele vacated the saloon of the ambulance and sat in the cab, waiting for the go ahead from me. I made sure George had enough blankets and was warm and comfortable, and also that he and his wife were safely strapped in.

'OK Adele, when you're ready!' I shouted. She turned the ignition, revved the engine, took the handbrake off and simultaneously tried to find the bite point between the accelerator and clutch, but there was no movement. 'When you're ready, Adele!' I repeated, thinking she hadn't heard me. There was still no movement.

'Andy!' Adele shouted. I got out of my seat and popped my head through the open, sliding glass window that separates the cab from the saloon.

'What's up?' I asked.

'The ambo's stuck, it won't move!' she informed me.

'Shit!' I thought, but quietly said, 'You are joking, aren't you? Please tell me you've just got a sick sense of humour.' That wouldn't have surprised me; paramedics tend to have just that, often worse than sick – dark and twisted in fact!

'No, I'm not joking, it won't move,' she said. My mind began to race. George needed to get to hospital as soon as possible, as the doctors would need to administer a subsequent dose of heparin to him through a drip a short time after receiving pre-hospital TNK. They also needed to obtain blood samples and undertake further ECGs to see whether the clot-busting drug had been successful or not.

'Right, jump in the back, I'll have a look outside,' I said to Adele.

She got out of the cab and entered the vehicle's saloon, while I stepped out and had a look at the position we were in. On inspection, it became apparent that we were stuck because the heavily falling snow had accumulated around the wheels of the ambulance. It was then that it dawned on me that we wouldn't be able to move without some help. I stepped back into the rear of the ambulance and said to Adele,

'We're going nowhere. I'm gonna contact Control and ask them to send another crew, or if none are available to attend immediately, then send the traffic police instead.'

If another crew was available, we would simply transfer George into their ambulance and they would convey him to hospital. Failing that, as the traffic police carry shovels for scooping up glass, car debris, eyeballs and other body parts from road traffic collisions, waiting a short time for the police was the next best option. So that's what I did, explaining the situation to ambulance control, including the fact that I'd given George TNK, amongst a concoction of other drugs too. There was no additional crew available. So, as it was a dire emergency, I asked them to send the traffic police on blue lights, preferably a motorway Range Rover in case we needed pulling out of the snow. I also asked them to contact the CCU department and explain the delay to them.

With my request carried out, all that could be done was to wait and monitor George for any improving or deteriorating signs and symptoms. While I went outside to try to clear some of the snow with my feet and hands, Adele undertook further periodic measurements of George's blood pressure, and printed several more ECGs to analyse whether any post-administration of TNK improvements were evident.

Ten minutes went by before I saw blue flashing lights approaching from the distance. It was the traffic police. They hadn't come in a Range Rover, they'd come in a Volvo Estate.

Nevertheless, they carried shovels and that's all that mattered. When they rolled up on scene I liaised with them and explained the predicament we were in. They then rapidly began to clear snow from around the wheels of the ambulance with their trusty shovels. Meanwhile, I stepped back into the saloon of the ambulance to allow Adele to take her position back in the driver's seat.

While waiting for the snow to be cleared, I alternated my gaze between George, his wife and Adele sat in the cab. As the minutes passed, George began to look pale, sweaty and a little vacant. Then, to my horror, his eyes closed and he slumped to one side. The warning alarms rang out on the ECG monitor. George was in cardiac arrest!

'Oh shit!' I thought, but instead shouted, 'Adele, get in the back, quick!'

'Oh god, what's happening?! George... oh god, what's happened?!' his wife cried out. Ignoring her, I glanced at the ECG monitor and immediately recognised that George's heart had deteriorated into Ventricular Fibrillation (VF). Adrenaline hurtled through my veins as I dropped the back of the stretcher down so George was laid flat. Then, using the bottom of my closed fist in a downward motion, I rapidly applied a pre-cordial thump to George's chest. A pre-cordial thump is intended to mimic what a defibrillator does to the heart, with a lot less energy and effect but it does occasionally work if applied almost immediately after a patient has arrested. On this occasion, it didn't! Adele leapt into the ambulance from the side door while I was applying the defibrillator pads to George's chest.

'What's happened?' she asked.

'He's in VF, I'm gonna shock him. Get the bag and mask out will you,' I said in a fast tone, pre-empting that we might need it. I turned to George's distraught wife and said, 'Stay calm for me, OK, stay calm.'

That was easy for me to say, but not so easy or pleasant for a lady to see her husband die right in front of her very own eyes and then, in simple terms, be about to see him electrocuted. As oxygen is a combustible gas, I removed the oxygen mask from his face for safety purposes, then switched the dial on the monitor to 'pads' and immediately pressed the 'charge' button.

'Charging!' I said out loud as a warning. Seconds later, the audible warning sounds echoed around the ambulance, informing me as the user that the appropriate energy had charged. 'Charged, stand clear, I'm clear!' I pressed the 'shock' button. An electrical current passed through George's body, causing his torso to lift an inch or so off the stretcher, which was normal during defibrillation. However, to George's wife it was so traumatising that she let out an almighty scream that, with our backs to her, made me and Adele jump with fright. 'Jesus!' I thought, 'Don't do that! My heart is already trying to escape from inside my chest without any more of a fright, thank you very much.'

Immediately after applying the shock, Adele and I checked the monitor, and to our joy the rhythm was back to a perfusing rhythm compatible with life. Before I even had chance to check George's carotid pulse in his neck, his eyes opened. He was oblivious to what had just happened, and was curious as to why his wife was so upset. By now sweating a little, I let out a big sigh of relief and then raised the back of the stretcher, restoring it to a semi-recumbent position. Adele, also sweating and shaking, comforted George's distraught wife.

Due to George's brief encounter with the afterlife, I printed another ECG and measured his blood pressure, while explaining to him what had just happened. To no surprise, he was shocked (pardon the pun) by my explanation of events.

What had happened to George can occur following the administering of TNK, although it hadn't happened before to other patients I'd thrombolysed, so it had taken me a little by surprise. However, it had been emphasised during thrombolysis training that whenever the drug actually achieves its purpose – i.e. successfully destroys a clot in the coronary artery – it causes an increase in oxygen delivery (reperfusion) to the heart muscle which can sometimes cause the heart to go in to an arrhythmia – in George's case, VF. The reason a single 'shock' restored his heart to a rhythm compatible with life, and also him becoming immediately conscious, was because defibrillation was carried out within seconds of him arresting. It is seldom successful if there is any considerable delay in defibrillating a patient who has been in a VF cardiac arrest for more than a few minutes, which is why pre-hospital cardiac arrest statistics are, unfortunately, very poor.

I learnt from that experience, and so I now place the defibrillation pads on all patients who are having a heart attack – in fact any patient who is at risk of deteriorating in to cardiac arrest – thus preventing any delay in 'shocking' the patient due to time spent applying the pads.

With normality restored, George's wife asked if her husband was going to be alright. I had to be honest with her and so tactfully explained that we needed to get him to hospital as fast as possible in order to increase his chance of survival in the long-term. Adele liaised with the police officers for a brief moment and then took her position back in the driver's seat and I gave her the all clear to move off. She revved the engine, took the handbrake off and found the bite between the accelerator and the clutch, and fortunately the vehicle moved away from the side of the road. Adele waved at the cavalry as she drove off,

'Thank you!' she shouted out of the window. The police were completely unaware of what had happened moments before.

Progressing slowly along the road towards the hospital, I closely monitored George's vital signs, including his ECG rhythm, and periodically comforted George's distraught wife at the same time. What appeared on the ECG was encouraging; the signs of a heart attack were gradually reducing. Thankfully, the drug was serving its purpose. George's pain score had by now reduced to a zero due to the analgesia administered and the clot-busting drug having a positive effect on the flow of oxygen to his heart. His colour had also improved and he had become a lot less sweaty and clammy, and George's facial expression appeared to show that of a man who wasn't so frightened anymore. The treatment administered was having a positive effect all round.

When we arrived at the CCU department, Adele promptly vacated the cab, opened the rear doors and lowered the ramp. We quickly wheeled the stretcher into the ward, followed by George's upset wife. She was escorted by a nurse to the waiting area where a patient's loved ones are expected to wait for good or bad news from the doctors. Meanwhile, I gave a handover to the awaiting consultant.

As paramedics are usually the first health care professionals on scene and hold vital information about an incident, a doctor usually listens to a handover from the paramedic while other doctors commence the assessment and treatment of the sick or injured patient. A handover is intended to summarise the history of events and observations undertaken by the paramedic, and the treatment provided. It is not usually conveyed grammatically or in full sentences, because doing so prolongs the process; if you have requested the resuscitation room, or in this case the CCU department, to be on standby, then the doctor needs information fast! Therefore, a handover is usually passed without interruption from anyone else in the room. For the benefit of the layperson, I have simplified handovers, where appropriate, throughout this book.

As we transferred George over to the hospital bed, I began my ungrammatical handover to the attentive doctor, which went something like this:

'This is George; he's fifty-seven years old and an insulin dependent diabetic. George was woken by central chest pain radiating down his left arm and into his jaw, at about two a.m. On arrival, he was fully conscious, breathing shallow and was anxious. He was ashen in colour, sweating profusely, clammy to the touch and complained of a pain score of ten, which he had experienced for approximately one hour by the time we had arrived at his side.

'Entonox initially administered, to some relief, and an aspirin was given too. George had a weak, slow pulse and an initial systolic blood pressure of one hundred, so GTN withheld, due to an unconfirmed heart attack in the lower portion of the heart.

'On further examination, his heart rate was thirty-three beats per minute. BP reduced to eighty systolic. His blood glucose was twenty-two, and his twelve lead ECG displayed signs of a heart attack.

30

'IV access obtained and five hundred micrograms of atropine administered to good effect. Heart rate increased to fifty-seven and systolic blood pressure increased to one hundred and ten, so a dose of GTN administered.

'George met all of the criteria for thrombolysis, so post atropine he received metoclopramide, morphine, heparin and TNK, but during the delay on scene deteriorated in to a VF arrest. A precordial thump was applied and a single shock was delivered. George immediately regained consciousness and was oblivious to the event.

'Further ECGs undertaken, and the most current is showing an improvement in heart tissue perfusion. Current pain score zero out of ten. Are there any questions?'

'No, thank you,' the doctor replied.

The CCU staff then continued with George's assessment, undertaking further post-thrombolysis observations on him. Adele and I went back out to the ambulance for some much needed fresh air. It was a relief to have got George into hospital alive, although he wasn't completely out of the woods yet, as the saying goes. He had a high chance of going in to cardiac arrest again at any time, until the occlusion in his coronary artery had completely dispersed or, as mentioned earlier, PPCI had been performed by surgeons.

After completing my documentation detailing the events that had occurred, Adele and I informed ambulance control that we were clear from hospital, and so we returned to station for a brew.

The following night, while at the same hospital and once again working with Adele, we decided to visit George in the CCU department before it got too late. Before visiting him at his bedside, I asked a duty nurse how George was. She informed me that thrombolysis had been successful and that he'd received PPCI too and was on the road to recovery, which was music to my ears given the predicament we had been in the previous night. After speaking with the nurse, Adele and I approached George, who was sat up in bed relaxing. He looked a picture of health compared to the previous night. He clearly remembered both of us and offered us his hand, and at the same time said,

'Thank you both for saving my life last night.'

'You're welcome,' I replied. 'But can I ask you a question out of intrigue; well, more so morbid curiosity really?'

'Of course,' he said.

'You know you hear stories about people in cardiac arrest looking down on themselves, say for instance, from the corner of a room, being resuscitated by medics and lay people, etcetera?'

'Yeah,' he replied, nodding his head.

'Well, did you see "the light"?' I asked, using flexed index and middle fingers of my hands to emphasise quotation marks. 'Or did you experience seeing any deceased relatives that told you to go back because it's not your time yet, or anything else?'

'No, nothing, just blackout, that's it,' he replied.

Chapter 2
Fighting a Losing Battle

During my career in the NHS Ambulance Service, I've worked alongside some exceptional health care professionals, including Consultants, GPs, Nurses, Auxiliaries, Paramedics, Ambulance Technicians, Emergency Care Assistants (or equivalent), and last but not least, those in other specialised professions such as Midwives, Radiographers and Physiotherapists, etcetera; all of whom had a high standard of patient care delivery at the forefront of their minds. However, targets set by the British Government often stand in the way of health care professionals providing the standard of patient care that they would wish to deliver.

I'm not having a rant; NHS politics aside, I'm still passionate about the job I do, and I want to do the best I can for my patients, as do most of my fellow professionals. I simply want to inform those who value their life and the lives of their loved ones, what goes on without your knowledge, and what could ultimately affect you or your loved ones as potential NHS patients.

Take the following for example: ambulances having to arrive on scene within eight minutes from call commencement to seventy-five percent of calls triaged as category 'A' life-threatening RED. My issue with this is that in a very, very high percentage of incidences where the patient is triaged as possessing life-threatening signs and symptoms, they are no closer to pushing daisies than I am of being the next *Stephen King*. That's right, nowhere near close! The call has simply been triaged inappropriately, following scripted questioning. What's more, if it takes the crew nine minutes to arrive on scene and they find that the patient is, as stated above, nowhere near to pushing daisies, then it is still audited as a missed category 'A' life-threatening RED call anyway. Madness!

In relation to the above, what is even more infuriating for frontline ambulance personnel is that, if they arrive on scene to attend to a patient with a genuine life-threatening illness or injury within eight minutes but the patient subsequently dies, it's not an issue; they'll hear nothing more about it because the target was achieved. Conversely, if an ambulance crew arrives on scene in ten minutes but manages to save a life, it is questioned, possibly even formally investigated as to why it took the crew that long. It all seems to be about targets and not about the quality of patient care or patient outcome.

The accuracy of triaging isn't down to ambulance control room call-takers. Oh no. It's the software used in the ambulance service around the UK to triage treble-nine and treble-one calls that is responsible. Although a variety of different software providers are contracted by the NHS, every system has been designed to triage the priority of response required based on the answers given by the caller to the questions asked by the call-taker. However, the non-human, automated aspect of the software prevents calls from being triaged appropriately.

For example, during a treble-one call – let's say a sixteen year old having a mild anxiety episode – the call-taker will ask if the patient they're calling about is short of breath. As one of the many side effects of an anxiety episode is shortness of breath, the caller will more often than not answer yes. The call-taker can then choose to skip further questioning and default to dispatching an emergency ambulance (which is often the case), or alternatively continue with further scripted questioning and wait to see what the software decides is the most suitable care pathway for the patient. However, despite further scripted questioning, the software will triage the said sixteen year old patient's condition as life-threatening. What started as a treble-one call is upgraded to a category 'A' life-threatening RED call that warrants a response within eight minutes from call commencement.

So, for the reasons outlined above, personnel of the modern day UK ambulance service are frequently responding to incidences under emergency driving conditions – which carries significant risk to life every time – only to find patients complaining of non-traumatic neck pain, a headache, or even a patient who has had chronic back pain for over twelve months! And many more symptoms that *do not* warrant an ambulance response at all, let alone a timely response. They're more often than not mere minor ailments that could be appropriately dealt with either by the patient's own GP or, more to the point, by oneself at home or following self-conveyance to an A&E department. If a medically trained person was solely responsible for triaging treble-nine and treble-one calls, as opposed to a non-human, automated software system, then more ambulance crews would be readily available for patients who *really* need an emergency ambulance.

My second example is A&E departments having to admit, transfer or discharge a patient within four hours of them arriving on the ward. Regardless of how professional and thorough the nurses and doctors wish to perform, having targets to achieve can cause patient assessment to be partial, or alternatively, complete but undertaken in a hurried manner. Unfortunately, due to the pressure placed on nurses and doctors, the patient is *sometimes* misdiagnosed as a consequence of achieving a four-hour turnaround. This can result in the patient being prematurely discharged and deteriorating while at home over the following two to forty-eight hours. Thus, an ambulance is called once again and the patient is brought back into the A&E department, and the whole process begins for a second time. Would you say that is *acting in the best interests of the patient*?

To act in the best interests of patients at all times is one of the many standards that health care professionals agree to adhere to when they apply for, or renew, their professional registration. However, that agreement is not always adhered to for one reason or another, but most often due to trying to achieve government targets. Now, while I don't entirely disagree with a four-hour turnaround target time, I do take issue that if a patient's condition is not serious or life-threatening, then why should doctors and nurses rush their assessments and treatment of those with more complex signs, symptoms and conditions just so uncompromised patients don't have to wait more than four hours to be attended to?

That brings me to this next incident, which involved mistakes being made by NHS staff due to the constant and relentless pressure they were under to achieve non-A&E (i.e. ward-based) government targets; an incident that ultimately landed me in court – Coroners Court, that is. Allow me to explain in great detail.

I was working a day shift as a solo responder on a Rapid Response Vehicle (RRV). It had been quite a busy day for me and the other crews from the station I was working at on this particular day. At 5 p.m. the RRV cab radio sounded.

'Go ahead, over,' I said.

'Roger, RED call to a sixty-seven year old male, collapsed but conscious, over,' the dispatcher said.

'Roger, understood, going mobile, over,' I replied, before activating my blue lights and sirens and mobilising in the direction of the address given.

When dispatched to a patient who has 'collapsed', the diagnosis could be anything from a heart attack or cardiac arrest, to fainting or simply being under the influence of alcohol or drugs. It might even be an unwitnessed trip or fall and not strictly a collapse. With my foot down, I arrived on scene within seven minutes. I vacated the RRV and grabbed the paramedic bag, oxygen bag and the ECG monitor from the saloon, then walked in haste down the garden pathway towards the wide open front door. A lady, who I rightly assumed was the patient's daughter, was stood in the doorway anticipating my arrival. She looked upset and was displaying signs of panic and angst.

'Hiya, my name's Andy, I'm a paramedic. What's the concern?' I asked while entering the premises.

'I don't know what's wrong, he just collapsed and he's complaining of abdominal pain, please help,' she said in a grief-stricken manner.

I could hear the sounds of someone retching and in agonising pain, coming from a room at the end of the hallway, so I moved fast towards the cries, which I then found were coming from the kitchen. I didn't know what to expect, in spite of the audible groans of pain I could hear, but when I arrived at the entrance to the kitchen, I was presented with nothing far short of the living dead! The elderly man, my patient, was laying on the tiled floor on his side, in the foetal position, agitated, holding his stomach with both hands and rolling back and forth in absolute agony. His face was a light shade of grey. His eyes intermittently opened and closed.

I immediately suspected something sinister was occurring, and that he was time-critical and only minutes from death. Crouching down beside him and placing my equipment within easy reach, I unzipped the pockets of the bag and began removing equipment, while at the same time questioning his distressed daughter.

'What's your name, my love?' I asked.

'Jan,' she informed me, with an evident look of concern on her face.

'OK Jan, stay calm for me. Now, what's your dad's name?'

'Jack,' she replied.

'And when did he collapse?'

'About ten minutes ago.'

Due to Jack's presentation, I immediately contacted ambulance control before I commenced any form of physical assessment. Jan was still stood close by, so I had to be careful of what I said.

'Requesting priority speech, over,' I said with assertion, and a little breathless from the sudden effects of adrenaline.

'Receiving, pass your priority, over,' the dispatcher said.

'Roger, I need immediate back-up. Patient collapsed, conscious but peri-arrest, over.' In the background, Jack's expression of pain and his retching sounded over my voice.

'Sorry, repeat your last, over,' the dispatcher said.

'Roger, I said I need immediate back-up. Patient collapsed, conscious but peri-arrest, over.'

'Roger, a crew has already been dispatched to you, over.'

'No divert!' I instructed, meaning under no circumstances send the ambulance en route to any other emergency call the dispatcher received in the meantime.

Peri-arrest is a medical term used to describe a patient who is potentially only minutes from cardiac arrest if lifesaving interventions are not undertaken swiftly. I knew the dispatcher wouldn't divert the crew, because she knew exactly what I meant by the term peri-arrest, but I wanted to make absolutely sure she understood my request and that it was logged on a recorded server. Fortunately, Jan didn't understand the terminology, which is what I'd hoped, as it may have caused her to panic even more.

Knelt down on the floor, with Jack by my side still rolling back and forth in the foetal position, I began assessing him. He was maintaining his own airway, and was evidently breathing as he was screaming out in pain. A time-critical patient who feels pain is a good sign, from a clinician's point of view, not from a patient's perspective, obviously. But if a seriously ill patient in severe pain becomes quiet without having any form of analgesia administered to them, whether pharmacological, distractional or positional, then that is not a good sign whatsoever, as it usually means they're worsening or have deteriorated in to cardiac arrest. I felt for a pulse in his right wrist. He had one. 'That's something at least,' I thought. I grabbed the SP02 monitor and placed it on an index finger. I waited for a moment, then a measurement displayed. Jack's sats were 85%, which was extremely poor. Due to his sats measurement, I grabbed an oxygen mask and hurriedly removed the plastic packaging, connected the tubing to the oxygen cylinder and placed the mask over his face, securing it with the elastic strap. Then I immediately administered high flow oxygen to him. Unfortunately, he was so anxious that he kept trying to grab it and pull it away from his face, while crying out in agony.

Jan was still very distressed and by now pacing about the kitchen, looking on, so I tried to distract her from what I was doing, which was preparing the defibrillation pads and unbuttoning Jack's shirt. Although difficult due to his agitation, I managed to apply the pads in their appropriate positions. That enabled me to monitor his heart rate, and would also prevent any delay in me administering a 'shock' if that became appropriate. While Jack lay on the floor, his pain continuing to be alarmingly evident as he screamed and retched, I ascertained some history from Jan.

'What's your dad's past medical history, Jan? He's grabbing his stomach, does he have abdominal problems?'

'He had abdominal surgery on his stomach ulcers six weeks ago, and he had a heart attack while on the ward. He died but he was resuscitated,' she said.

Mentioning stomach ulcers concerned me as he was grey in colour, and the heart rate on the monitor was displaying 140 BPM. I started to think an internal bleed was highly likely. Pre-empting that a cardiac arrest was about to ensue, I turned to Jan and said,

'Look, this isn't pleasant for you to see, so if you want to leave the room then that's fine by me.'

'OK, I'll go to a neighbour's house then, a close friend of my dad's, and let 'em know he's going back into hospital,' she said, extremely upset. But as she was walking down the hallway towards the front door, it suddenly dawned on me: 'What if he arrests while she's gone?' On that thought, I shouted,

'Jan!' She returned to the kitchen. 'Just let your dad know where you're going. And tell him that you love him, OK. I'll do my best, and I've got more help on the way.'

Stood by her dad, tears running down her face, Jan leant over and said,
'Dad, it's Jan. I'm going to Harry's to let him know you're going to hospital, OK? I love you, won't be long.' Jack didn't acknowledge Jan's message, he just continued to writhe around in agony.

I'd been on scene for just a couple of minutes but had swiftly suspected that I was dealing with an internal bleed. So my next thought was, 'Get IV access and get some fluid up quick! It might just buy him some time.' I held Jack's wrist and assertively asked him to let go of his stomach, which he did, after some gentle persuasion. I then applied a tourniquet to his left arm, chose a large bore cannula from the paramedic bag and waited for a viable vein to appear. After a minute or so of waiting, to my disappointment, no blue tinge had appeared. 'This is not looking good,' I thought. I could have tried the other arm but instead chose to attempt cannulating an area of his arm where a vein should physiologically be. I prepared a cannula and held it in my right hand, holding his arm with my left. I pierced the skin with the needle and waited for the flashback of blood to appear in the chamber, which usually means successful IV access. But there was no flashback.

'Shit!' I said openly, as there was no one else around other than Jack, and it was unlikely that he would have heard it over his agonising cries. With no flashback evident, I chose to manipulate the needle a little, hoping that doing so would prove successful. It wasn't. There was no viable vein, he was far too shutdown. I removed the tourniquet from around his arm and placed it onto the floor on his right side, with the intention of making a second attempt, on his right arm, a minute or so later. I discarded the needle into the sharps container and quickly applied a small dressing to the puncture wound.

With Jack still conscious but agitated and writhing around in agony, I wrapped the automatic blood pressure cuff around his right arm and pressed the start button. While the monitor was analysing his blood pressure, I removed the BVM (bag-valve-mask), used to ventilate patients, from the paramedic bag and placed it alongside Jack's head, along with some airway adjuncts and a manual suction device used to suction various fluids, including vomit, from the airway. Sweat was by now running down my face onto the hard kitchen floor, and my gloved hands were wringing wet through. I felt like pulling my gloves off and washing my hands in the nearby sink before I got back to work, but time was of the essence. I needed IV access so I could get some fluid up and try to prevent Jack from deteriorating in to cardiac arrest, if at all possible.

While I was preparing equipment for a second attempt at cannulation, Jack's audible cries of pain reduced slightly, over thirty seconds or so, and the speed and repetitiveness of him rolling back and forth also decreased. His hands gradually loosened from around his stomach, and a gurgling sound emerged from his mouth, as if taking his last breath. Then he went limp and quiet. No more cries of agonising pain.

'Jack! Jack!' I shouted. I looked at the ECG monitor, 'Shit!' His heart rate had changed from the 140 BPM displayed since applying the pads on my arrival, to zero BPM. That's a 'flatline' to the layperson. As anticipated, Jack had abruptly deteriorated in to cardiac arrest!

I rapidly moved to the head end of Jack's body laid motionless on the tiled floor and palpated for a pulse in his neck, just in case it was a fault with the machine: *Treat the patient, not the machine*, as they say in the medical profession. There was no pulse. The machine had correctly interpreted Jack's heart rhythm; it was definitely a flatline. So, knelt at Jack's head end and using open speech on the hand portable radio, I contacted ambulance control.

'Requesting priority speech, over,' I said in an abrupt tone. Simultaneously, with my free hand, I began compressing Jack's chest at a rate of one hundred times per minute. One-handed is less effective on an adult but better than doing no chest compressions at all.

'Roger, pass your priority, over,' the dispatcher said.

'Roger, this is now a cardiac arrest. ETA on back-up?' I said, panting a little from the exertion of chest compressions and an increase in adrenaline. Using the satellite tracking device to locate the back-up vehicle, the controller came back to me and said,

'Roger, they're about five minutes away, over.'

'Roger.'

After the very short radio conversation was over, I temporarily ceased compressions, removed the oxygen mask from Jack's face, extended his neck and inserted an oral adjunct into his mouth to afford him a patent airway. I attached the BVM tubing to the oxygen cylinder and ventilated him with two squeezes of the bag, before recommencing compressions.

I sustained compressions and periodic ventilations for two minutes, before ceasing in order to check the monitor for any change in the rhythm of his heart. There was no change. So I carried on with the Basic Life Support (BLS) algorithm while I waited for the back-up crew to arrive. My plan was to progress to the Advanced Life Support (ALS) algorithm upon their arrival, which would involve obtaining a definitive airway by intubating Jack – that is, placing a tube down his windpipe and then inflating a balloon on the tube. That would prevent any regurgitated gastric contents from entering his lungs. The ALS algorithm would also involve having another attempt at gaining IV access and administering drugs and fluid.

While ventilating Jack, more gurgling sounds emerged from his mouth with each squeeze, so I ceased ventilating and checked his airway. To my alarm, blood had begun to accumulate in his mouth. So, swiftly grabbing the manual suction device, I began suctioning the blood from his airway, collecting the claret in the container attached. I then provided two more ventilations with the BVM before recommencing chest compressions. A minute or so later, I heard sirens close by. 'Excellent, they're here,' I thought. To my relief, a short time later, the crew entered the house.

'Andy!' Alf, a paramedic, shouted.

'I'm in the kitchen, but get me the automatic suction and another oxy cylinder will you, mate!' Alf then shouted to his technician crewmate, Gemma, to bring the equipment that I'd requested, and then proceeded into the kitchen to assist me.

'What have we got, mate?' he asked, taking over chest compressions.

'Right, this is Jack, I found him collapsed, evidently suffering with abdominal pain. He was peri-arrest on my arrival, then he arrested about five minutes ago. He keeps regurgitating blood, so I think the cause of his arrest is a massive internal bleed. I need to suction and get a tube in quick,' I said, while using the manual suction device to remove more blood from Jack's airway.

'OK, mate. Did you get IV access before he arrested?' Alf asked.

'No, I missed on his left side. When Gemma comes in, you have a go on his right arm while I tube him.'

'Yeah, OK,' Alf replied.

Gemma entered the kitchen and passed me another full oxygen cylinder and the automatic suction machine, which has a more powerful 'vacuum' than a manual device. Glancing at Gemma, I said,

'Can you put all the equipment I need to intubate next to me, and then take over chest compressions while Alf has a go at IV access?' While Gemma did as I had asked, I suctioned some more blood from Jack's airway and then continued with periodic ventilations.

Gemma had placed the appropriate equipment beside me and had taken over compressions. Her responsibility would be to stop compressions every two minutes and check whether the

ECG monitor was displaying a change in cardiac rhythm. Alf, on the other hand, was having difficulty gaining IV access. Unfortunately, no viable vein appeared in Jack's right arm. After attempting to cannulate where a vein should physiologically have been, as I had, he missed and so had to withdraw the needle, patch up the wound and cease attempts, for the time being anyway.

It is worth me mentioning that since the time this incident occurred, paramedics have been trained and equipped to undertake intraosseous (IO) access – 'osseous' referring to bone. IO access is achieved by literally drilling a cannula into the bone of the shin or shoulder. It is not necessarily paramedics' preferred or primary choice of access – that is, with the exception of a paediatric cardiac arrest, where veins are rarely visible – but provides a secondary option in the event IV access cannot be achieved.

After suctioning yet more blood from Jack's airway, I informed Gemma that I was ready to attempt intubation and asked her to stop compressions, so the movement of the body didn't obscure my view of his vocal chords. I held the laryngoscope – used to shift the tongue to the left – in my left hand, with an appropriately sized tube in my right, and then placed the laryngoscope into Jack's mouth and attempted to view his vocal chords. As I was doing that, blood began to fill his airway again. That obscured my view and made intubation at that time impossible. So I withdrew the laryngoscope and asked Gemma to continue with compressions, before suctioning Jack's airway once again. But his airway almost immediately filled with blood again, before I even had chance to insert the laryngoscope into his mouth.

My heart was thumping against my chest because of the frustration and the difficult predicament I was in. Without a patent airway, free of contents – in this case blood – we were fighting a losing battle and there would be absolutely no hope whatsoever of saving Jack's life! His blood-filled airway would have been a challenge for an anaesthetist, I'm sure. Having said that, I don't want to do anaesthetists an injustice there; *they* may have found it really easy – they are airway management experts, after all. Then again, with the obvious exception of emergency surgery, their patients are usually *nil by mouth* for twelve to twenty-four hours and are only likely to regurgitate blood during an operation and after they've already been anaesthetised and intubated.

With Jack's airway by now constantly accumulating blood, and me flushed and with beads of sweat dripping off my forehead and face, I turned to the crew and said,

'It's no good. Gemma, continue with compressions until I'm ready to 'ave another go. Alf, it's gonna take two of us, mate.'

'OK, what do you wanna do?' Alf asked.

'Right, you suction while I try and intubate. It's gonna be difficult, but it's our only option,' I said to Alf while simultaneously ventilating Jack and looking at the collecting bag of the suction device. Blood was now at the level of four hundred millilitres.

Alf positioned himself next to me and suctioned blood from Jack's mouth. With compressions ceased, I prepared myself for what was going to have to be a rapid attempt at securing a tube in place. So, as knelt down as I could possibly be, I lifted his tongue to the left with the laryngoscope.

'I can see the chords,' I said, thinking out loud. Blood began to accumulate again. 'Alf, suction, quick!' Alf provided a little more suction. The chords were in view again, so in haste but carefully I attempted to position the tube. Blood rapidly filled his airway, quicker than I could place the tube through the correct landmark. 'Suction again, Alf!' I shouted. Alf did as I asked, and as he suctioned I rapidly inserted the tube through the visible vocal chords and into Jack's windpipe. 'I'm in! Gemma, continue with compressions. Alf, inflate the balloon!' He pressed the pre-positioned syringe attached to the tube, causing the balloon to inflate, thus preventing any more blood from entering Jack's lungs. Alf then took hold of the tube, stopping it from becoming displaced.

I asked Gemma to cease compressions for a moment while I placed my stethoscope over various positions on Jack's chest to listen to his lung fields. At the same time, I squeezed the ventilating bag attached to the end of the tube, to ensure correct placement. Happy that it was correctly placed, I secured it by tying a net-like bandage around the tube and then around Jack's face and head. Alf attached the automatic ventilator, which meant that Jack was being ventilated hands-free. Gemma was now able to perform chest compressions non-stop, with the exception of briefly checking the monitor every two minutes for any change in heart rhythm.

Both Alf and I had attempted IV access on each of Jack's arms, albeit without success, so the next option was to cannulate his jugular vein in his neck. While Jack was being automatically ventilated, and compressions were being performed by Gemma, I turned his head to one side, hoping that a jugular vein would reveal itself. It did. It was extremely poor but enough to attempt external jugular cannulation (EJC). Alf passed me a cannula, so I quickly removed the packaging and inserted the cannula into the vein in Jack's neck, before flushing it with a little sodium chloride and securing it in place with an adhesive dressing. With IV access secured, Alf passed me both a pre-filled syringe of adrenaline and of atropine. I immediately administered one drug after the other. Meanwhile, Alf had begun to prepare a bag of fluid in order to replace some of the fluid volume that Jack had lost, and continued to lose, internally from somewhere in his stomach.

Gemma continued to perform chest compressions, as the automatic ventilator continued to provide ventilations. Other than to administer periodic adrenaline to Jack, there was nothing else we could do until his heart rhythm converted to a rhythm compatible with life, or to a 'shockable' rhythm where defibrillation would then be indicated. Alas, a patient with an internal bleed is unlikely to present with, or develop, a 'shockable' rhythm post cardiac arrest.

Alf took over compressions from Gemma to give her a rest. While he was doing that, I heard someone stepping through the front door, so I immediately went out to the hallway to see who it was. It was Jan. She instantly knew that something was wrong, and so I tactfully and sympathetically informed her that after she had left, her dad deteriorated further and subsequently arrested, but we were attempting to resuscitate him. Understandably, she sobbed her heart out. Choosing not to witness or experience her dad being resuscitated, she went into the lounge and made a phone call to her mum, Jack's wife, who was unaware of the tragic occurrences that had unfolded a short time before.

Resuscitation continued for a further ten minutes, and by now Jack had been 'down' for over twenty minutes with no change in ECG rhythm. The ECG monitor still displayed a flatline. There were no clinical signs that he was making any respiratory effort, no evidence of a return of spontaneous circulation – that is, a pulse – and his pupils were fixed and dilated. Sadly, Jack was not responding to treatment... he was dead.

We had to accept that he was gone and no amount of CPR was going to bring him back. So Gemma, Alf and I all agreed that resuscitation should be stopped. I switched the ventilator off and closed the pinch on the fluid giving set, and Gemma ceased performing chest compressions. I looked at the collecting bag of the suction device and there was half a litre of blood inside it. I couldn't believe how much had been suctioned from Jack's airway. And in view of the difficult airway management that I'd experienced, he probably had accumulations of blood in his lungs and a bucket full in his stomach too. Prior to attending to Jack, I hadn't suctioned that amount of blood from a patient's airway, and haven't seen the like of it right up to the time of writing this account.

At the time of ceasing resuscitation, I didn't know what the exact cause was, and didn't expect to find out for some time, if ever. We all came to our feet and Alf and Gemma began clearing up all the mess that we had made. Meanwhile, I went into the lounge to deliver the heartbreaking news to Jan. I informed her that after over twenty minutes of resuscitation, her dad had not responded to treatment and sadly I had confirmed him dead. Understandably, she was absolutely devastated to say the least.

After I'd helped Gemma and Alf clear up, they vacated the

premises and began their return journey to the ambulance station. I'd informed ambulance control of the time of death and they had notified the police, who would attend the scene to act on behalf of the coroner's office. By then Jan had made some further telephone calls to members of her family. A short time later, Jack's wife arrived home, extremely distressed, and then further family members began to arrive too. They were shocked, because Jack had been successfully resuscitated in hospital just several weeks prior, so the family had been very hopeful. They certainly hadn't expected that Jack's life would be over so soon after being discharged.

While sat in the lounge with the family, completing the appropriate paperwork and waiting for the police to arrive, I began ascertaining Jack's past medical history in more detail. Upon being educated by his wife regarding the medication Jack had been on, I learnt something that prompted me to raise my eyebrows, figuratively speaking. Now, I'm no pharmacist or doctor, far from it – I'm a *Jack of All Trades, Master of None*, remember? – but to what was my knowledge at the time, the three particular drugs that Jack had been prescribed should not have been ingested together by anybody, not just Jack. I believed his medication would most certainly have caused, or played a significant role, in his death. I chose to say nothing to the family about my suspicions and instead decided to keep my limited knowledge to myself, as it would have been very unprofessional of me if I was wrong. Nevertheless, I anticipated a request to attend Coroner's Court in the distant future.

After spending some time completing the paperwork, discussing with the police what had happened, giving Jack's family my sympathies, and having apologised several times for us not being able to do more for him, I vacated the premises and returned to the ambulance station to restock equipment.

Several months later, as predicted, I was told that the HM Coroner had requested a witness statement from me. He wanted a detailed explanation of the events that unfolded on that particular day I attended to Jack. Alf and Gemma did not need to write a statement or attend court, one of us was enough. Witness statements for the coroner have to be formally written and are therefore usually time consuming to write, edit and rewrite. The statement has to include your full name and how long you have been a paramedic. It also has to be double spaced and typed using an appropriately sized, legible font. So I spent two days recalling and documenting the events of that day, and by the time I was happy that my statement was an accurate account of my version of events, it totalled nine pages of A4 paper. I returned my statement and awaited a date to attend Coroner's Court.

That day came several months later (they don't rush these things), and I'd obviously been stood down from duty to attend court. Upon waking up that morning, I immediately felt nervous and apprehensive, even though I wasn't expecting to be scrutinised by the coroner. I would be there to explain the circumstances I'd been presented with on that day, and what my actions had been when I arrived at Jack's side. However, two NHS health care professionals were going to be scrutinised by the coroner because mistakes had been made, and I knew exactly what those mistakes had been, or at least I thought I did!

I'd pressed a clean uniform, had my hair cut and had brutally polished my boots the day before. I also ensured that I had a close, clean-cut shave that morning, and also applied an excessive amount of non-fragrant antiperspirant underneath my arms, as I'd anticipated that I was going to sweat profusely!

When I arrived at court, I was given a copy of my statement and asked to sit, along with others, and wait to be called to the stand. Even though so long had gone by since the incident, I immediately recognised Jan and other family members in the court room, including Jack's wife. They recognised me but made no friendly facial gesture. In fact, when they glanced at me it felt like they were angry at me, like I was to blame for Jack's death. That made me even more nervous, paranoid in fact, and I started to think that maybe I was going to be scrutinised by the coroner after all. I began asking myself all sorts of questions: 'Do the family think it was my fault he died, or that I gave up on him too soon? Do they think I should have done more? Did I put the tube in Jack's stomach instead of his windpipe and not realised it? No, I definitely correctly placed the tube, I'm sure.'

It was horrible sat in that court room, waiting for the coroner to arrive. Eventually, he entered.

'All stand,' the clerk instructed. We all stood, emphasising our respect for the HM Coroner… or for the Queen, I'm not sure. The Queen, I think. I was called as the first witness and so reluctantly walked to the stand and took an oath. I felt like I was on trial for murder. Regardless of the fact I'd sprayed half a can of antiperspirant underneath each armpit, sweat was still dripping down my torso, fortunately unnoticeable to everybody else in the court room.

The coroner usually undertakes a particular format when questioning a witness at an inquest. They either instruct you to read your statement out to everybody in the room, or *they* read it to everybody in the room. Or the statement isn't read out in full, the coroner merely questions the witness about pertinent parts of their statement. On this particular day, the coroner chose the latter, with me anyway. So he went through the events of that day, reciting parts of my statement to the attentive people in the court room, occasionally pausing to ask me if a particular part of the statement was correct. 'Of course it's correct, it's all correct, it's my statement, I wrote it,' I thought.

After forty minutes or so of grilling, the coroner told me I could step down. Then, to my horror, before I had chance to stand from the seat, the family solicitor asked the coroner if he could say a few words to me on behalf of the family. The coroner granted his request. The solicitor then directed his eyes at me and said,

'The family would like to thank you and your colleagues for your actions on that day, and the fact that you gave Jack the benefit of the doubt under such difficult circumstances; it couldn't have been easy or a pleasant experience for you and your colleagues, thank you.' I didn't know how to respond, so I just looked in the direction of the family, gently grinned and nodded my head at them. I stepped down from the stand and was escorted from the court room by the clerk.

Once outside of the room, I let out a huge sigh of relief. 'Thank god that is over! I'm never doing that again,' I thought. Yeah, right, like I should be so lucky!

Shortly after the inquest, I found out the exact mistakes that had been made by two doctors, and although my suspicions had not been entirely correct, I wasn't far off. The coroner's inquest highlighted that although the medication Jack had been prescribed *can* be taken together by some people, in Jack's case, due to his medical history of stomach ulcers, taking the drugs together was contraindicated for *him*. Ingesting all three of the medications together for several weeks caused him a massive internal bleed, with fatal consequences.

What had been the cause of contraindicative drugs being prescribed to Jack? A communication and documentation error between the two doctors who, as mentioned earlier, had been under constant and relentless pressure to achieve government targets. When under constant pressure mistakes are inevitable, sometimes to the detriment of patients' health and safety, or in this case the patient's life. Jack obviously wasn't the first patient to die due to health care professionals' errors, and he certainly wouldn't be the last.

Of course, I'm not suggesting that *all* errors are caused as a consequence of NHS staff attempting to achieve government targets. Health care professionals are only human after all, and *all* humans make mistakes. That's why there's a little eraser at the end of pencils, isn't it? Nevertheless, it is definitely safe to say that government targets do play a significant part in what could be preventable deaths, of that I am sure!

Unfortunately, I will never forget that incident for as long as I live. Fortunately, situations where a patient is going to die while in your care as a paramedic, with a family member present or close by, are few and far between. I knew Jack was going to die on me from the moment I arrived at his side. I could have, and in hindsight should have, been up front and honest with Jan and told her that her dad wasn't going to make it. At the time, I didn't know what the most ethical approach was: allow her to watch her dad writhe around in torturous pain and distress before dying in front of her, or persuade her to leave and miss what was the one and only opportunity she would ever get to say goodbye, and anything else she might have wanted to say. It was a difficult call to make, but I'm content and can sleep at night knowing that I had told her to tell him that she loved him, and that she had done so before he sadly passed away.

Chapter 3
A Logistical Nightmare

The modern day ambulance service is evolving; it has to, not only from a clinical point of view but in terms of fleet care and health and safety too. Why? Well, I don't know if you have noticed but in today's society people are becoming ever increasingly larger. As a result, NHS ambulance services have had to be involved in the design of bariatric ambulances – *bariatric* referring to treatment of the obese – to accommodate the increasing population of larger patients. And, I assume, all NHS staff have had and will continue to have further training in manual handling and lifting, to lessen their chance of sustaining a short or long-term injury, particularly a back injury. If further training and new equipment is not implemented then the number of staff absent from duty will be plentiful, and a significant reduction in fit, healthy and capable NHS staff would obviously affect the standard of patient care provided in the UK, both pre-hospital and in-hospital.

I once asked an NHS Trust Health and Safety Officer, while discussing the mixed subjects of back injuries, verbal abuse and violent assault on ambulance personnel, would she prefer to spend NHS money on back care or stab-proof vests for frontline ambulance crews? Her answer was back care, her reason being that ambulance personnel are more likely to be pensioned-off, or taken down the capability route, due to a chronic back injury than they are to be stabbed to death in the line of duty. At the time I took offence to her choice of prioritisation because, regardless that the likelihood of being stabbed while on duty was slim, it would only take one incident to justify *all* operational ambulance personnel wearing a stab-proof vest. During that conversation, it became apparent that it was worth taking the risk and not spend money on stab-proof vests, but instead allocate available funding to save ambulance personnel from suffering a back injury. In hindsight, I can see where she was coming from; she was bang on the button.

Over recent years, it has been widely reported in the national press and the media that the number of overweight and obese adults in the UK has been progressively increasing. Today, it is estimated that nearly half of men and one third of women in England are overweight. By overweight they are referring to having a Body Mass Index (BMI) of 25-30. It is also estimated that an additional one quarter of men and around one third of women are obese, that is they have a Body Mass Index of more than 30. A healthy Body Mass Index is between 20 and 24.9. The BMI formula is not without its flaws, granted, because it is calculated by using the subject's total weight in kilograms by their height in metres, squared. To put those flaws into context, if you imagine *Arnold Schwarzenegger* when he first won the 'tall' category of the Mr Universe Championships as an amateur in 1967, he would have been classed as obese. Umm, do you see my point? Nevertheless, despite the example of Arnie and the BMI formula's flaws, there is no doubt that we in the UK have become an overweight society.

Throughout my career in the ambulance service, I've attended to numerous obese patients; not overly frequently, though I have to admit it's becoming progressively more frequent. I once read an article on the subject of obesity and the consequential career span of future frontline ambulance personnel. It stated that, due to the ever increasing body size of today's society, those entering the paramedic profession *today* won't be fit enough to be frontline in ten years' time. That's a daunting thought – a mere ten year paramedical career before you're condemned to the 'useless heap' because of a back injury, or a torn rotator cuff injury, from lifting obese patients day in, day out. If lifting obese patients frequently is predicted to become the norm in the not too distant future, then I will certainly be pursuing a non-operational role, or leaving the ambulance service altogether!

Anyway, from the countless number of overweight and obese patients that I've attended to, there is one particular incident that springs to mind that I'll never forget, due to the sad circumstances surrounding the patient involved, as well as the unforeseen, undignified events that evolved while my crewmate and I, and another ambulance crew, attended to him.

I was on a twelve-hour day shift one bright, sunny morning, sat relaxing in the ambulance station with Carol, my crewmate. Carol had a fantastic sense of humour and I loved working with her because we always had a great laugh; sometimes, where appropriate, even while attending to a patient. I remember we once convinced a patient that we were a married couple, before we began to bicker in their presence. The patient, who was not in the least bit poorly and had no need to attend hospital, was in stitches watching us debate who was going to be doing the cooking that night. He was one of those patients, like many patients ambulance crews around the country attend to, that enjoyed a little banter and did not perceive our humour as unprofessional. If you're in the ambulance service and reading this, you'll understand what I mean; if you're not, you may think otherwise.

Carol and I had been on duty for a few hours when the RED call radio alarm sounded.

'Go ahead, over,' I said.

'Roger, RED call to back-up your crewmates who are in attendance of a thirty-nine year old male collapsed in respiratory arrest, over.'

'Roger, understood, over,' I replied.

By respiratory arrest, the dispatcher meant that the patient had a cardiac output – that is, a pulse – but he wasn't breathing. The best chance of survival and recovery is immediate and decisive treatment, which involves ventilating a patient using the BVM. Respiratory arrest often, not always, develops to a full cardiac arrest within minutes of occurring. So Carol and I vacated the ambulance station, boarded the ambulance and mobilised towards the address given.

En route, Carol and I queried why the crew would want back-up, as respiratory arrest could, in most cases, be easily dealt with as a double-manned crew and would normally be a 'scoop and run' incident, where the paramedic would provide the patient with assisted ventilations all the way to hospital, either by BVM or intubation and automatic ventilations.

We had only been mobile for a couple of minutes when the cab radio sounded. 'We're being stood down,' I thought. I was wrong! The dispatcher gave us an update which informed us that the patient was now in cardiac arrest. Even with that information, we were still unsure why the crew wanted back-up, as ambulance crews often deal with cardiac arrests as a two-man team, maybe three if an RRV is readily available to attend as well.

When we arrived on scene and vacated the ambulance cab, the reason the crew had requested back-up became very clear. While stood on the pavement and overlooking the low-bricked wall in to the patient's front garden, we were presented with a man-mountain laid flat on his back, with ECG pads applied to his chest. Jim, one of the crew members that had been first on scene, was knelt at the patient's head end, intermittently performing assisted ventilations and chest compressions. Due to the sheer size and obesity of the patient, Jim was evidently finding it difficult to perform chest compressions with an adequate and effective depth, thus being unable to afford sufficient circulation around the patient's body.

Also stood in the garden was the patient's wife. She appeared incredibly calm, given the unpleasant sight she was experiencing, but I think she was calm because she was unaware of the seriousness of the situation. Carol and I proceeded through the garden gate and approached Jim's crewmate, Tom, a paramedic. He was knelt beside the patient, looking for a potential vein to cannulate. I crouched down beside him.

'Hiya Andy, this is Rob, he collapsed in respiratory arrest but he's now in asystole. I can't find a vein though. We've got the fire service en route to assist us,' Tom said. Carol took over chest compressions from Jim to give him a rest, but he continued with intermittent assisted ventilations. However, because of Rob's enormity, Carol too was unable to provide an effective and adequate depth of compression.

With ineffective compressions, Rob's heart in a flatline rhythm and no fire service yet on scene to assist us to get Rob into the ambulance, resuscitation was futile. Despite that, we decided to do our utmost best for the sake of Rob's onlooking wife at least, to provide her with the peace of mind that we were doing our best to save her husband's life. While Jim and Carol periodically swapped resuscitative roles, I went and knelt down on Rob's left side and began to look for a vein in his left arm. While doing that, Tom discreetly informed me, in a low tone of voice and out of ears-reach of Rob's wife nearby, of the events leading up to him collapsing and the subsequent request for back-up.

He explained that Rob was forty to fifty-stone in weight and had not stepped outside, over the threshold of his front door, for over two years. He also informed me that he and Jim had initially been given the call as a patient with chest pain. Upon their arrival at Rob's side, they had ascertained a pertinent history and undertaken some baseline observations, including a 12-Lead ECG. Following that, they had suspected that Rob's condition was cardiac in nature and therefore potentially life-threatening, and so advised him to go to hospital. That is where the logistical problems arose, because the safe weight-load of the make and model carry-chair in use during this incident was nineteen stone, if I remember rightly. It may have been twenty-four stone; I can't recall for sure now because they've since been replaced with another model that can withstand a heavier weight-load. Anyway, at the time, Rob was around twice the weight of the safe load the carry-chair had been designed and manufactured to tolerate. Plus, the surface area of the chair hadn't been adequate for Rob to park his backside on.

So while they had still been in the lounge, Tom had tactfully explained to Rob that he was too heavy for the carry-chair and so asked if he could manage to walk the short distance from the lounge to the front door. He would then be able to rest on the carry-chair, but only for a short time as the metal frame of the chair might not have been able to sustain his weight for a prolonged period. Having a brief rest would at least enable him to inhale some Entonox before continuing to walk towards the ambulance. Rob had said he could but that he'd be very slow.

As an egress decision had been agreed, Tom had placed the carry-chair near the open front door. Rob had then stood from the armchair in the lounge and had slowly walked to the awaiting carry-chair but became breathless in the process; bearing in mind he still had chest pain irrespective of inhaling Entonox. After parking part of his backside on the carry-chair for a brief period before coming to his feet again, he proceeded to step over the threshold of the front door and had begun to amble across the front garden towards the waiting ambulance. But now stood in the garden, Rob had once again become breathless, so Tom placed the carry-chair onto the grass. Rob let the chair take his weight again and had another rest to get his breath back. However, while partially seated and resting, Rob took a turn for the worse and became so breathless that he collapsed from the carry-chair.

Rob had ceased breathing for himself. Tom and Jim had immediately intervened with assisted ventilations and requested ambulance and fire service back-up. Unfortunately, Rob's condition deteriorated to a cardiac arrest prior to Carol and I arriving. That was the history of events that had occurred, and how we'd come to arrive at the logistical nightmare we were all now experiencing. Rob had been 'down' in a flatline rhythm for some ten minutes when a fire appliance rolled up on scene.

As resuscitation continued, albeit ineffective and with no IV access obtained, the full complement of firemen joined us in the garden. Tom explained to them what had happened and the predicament that lay ahead of us. The dilemma was that Rob was now technically classed as 'deceased in a public place'. Yes, his own front garden. Normal ambulance service procedure is that if a patient is in a public place, they have to be moved even if resuscitation has ceased, or was not even commenced for one reason or another; for example, if rigor mortis (post death stiffening of the body) is present. The exception is in the case of suspicious circumstances. If that is the case then Scenes of Crime Officers (SoCO) would put a tent over the body while they investigate further. If resuscitation is undertaken in a patient's home and they're confirmed deceased, they're not removed from the house by the NHS ambulance service at all. Instead, the deceased is *usually* removed by a funeral director acting on behalf of the coroner's office.

The fire service brought a huge canvas sheet into the garden. The plan, as undignified as it was, was to place the sheet, folded concertina-like, on one side of Rob, then to literally roll him on to his side and pull a sufficient amount of the sheet underneath him. Following that, then to roll him a little more, until he was roughly in the middle of the canvas sheet.

As they prepared the sheet, I stood beside Rob's wife and explained what we were trying to do. During that explanation, she interrupted and said,

'Should I go and get his pyjamas in case they keep him in?'

Well, put yourself in that position, what would you have said to that? I chose to say what I thought was best at the time under the circumstances, so I replied with,

'No, don't worry about that right now.'

So, between the full complement of firemen, Tom, Jim, Carol

and I, we positioned the canvas sheet underneath Rob and were ready to attempt to lift him. Just as we were about to lift the canvas sheet off the ground with Rob in situ, further problems surfaced that we hadn't initially thought about. Firstly, we wouldn't be able to lift him high enough to place him on the stretcher. And secondly, even if we could lift him the height of the stretcher, he wasn't going to fit *on to* the stretcher... he would overhang the sides.

Unfortunately, we had no choice but to allow the whole incident to become even more undignified for Rob. We removed the stretcher from Tom and Jim's ambulance and placed it into the back of mine and Carol's ambulance. That left the entire floor space of their ambulance free to accommodate Rob's, yet to be officially confirmed deceased, body. Between us all, we grabbed a section of the canvas sheet, having had no choice but to cease resuscitation – which unavoidably reduced the already poor chance of a successful outcome – and lifted him off the floor. And when I say off the floor, it was barely an inch; he was so heavy we could hardly walk and lift at the same time.

We slowly progressed from the garden towards the gate, having then to squeeze him through it and place ourselves in awkward positions so we could keep lifting him and get through the gate ourselves. The weight caused our grip to gradually be prised open and made our fingers turn a shade of blue. Fortunately, while all that was happening, there weren't many pedestrians about or cars driving passed, although those that did pass naturally gawped. Two ambulances and a fire appliance parked outside of a house often causes people to gawp out of curiosity. Human nature, I suppose.

When we'd moved Rob through the gate and on to the roadside, we had to literally drag him up the fold-out steps of the ambulance, before placing him onto the floor. After we'd let go of the canvas sheet, vacated the ambulance and looked back in, Rob covered almost the entire available floor space; so much so that Tom, who was going to be travelling in the back with Rob to the hospital, had no room whatsoever to adopt a position suitable to allow him to continue resuscitation attempts. Not that continued resuscitation was going to make any difference to the outcome of Rob's condition; with basic life support attempts having been both interrupted and ineffective for a prolonged period, he was, unfortunately and without a doubt, dead!

With the back doors of the ambulance still open, I had a short discussion with Tom and we both agreed that we should inform Rob's wife that resuscitation had now ceased. So I slammed the back doors shut and approached Rob's wife and asked her to step inside the house. There, I broke the very sad news to her that her husband had died.

Now, I've not been counting but I imagine I've pronounced at least one thousand people dead during my career so far. Pronouncing that someone is dead is a frequent encounter for ambulance personnel and, with the exception of children and young adults, you get used to it: it may sound heartless to the layman but it becomes like water off a duck's back, particularly when the patient is elderly. However, having to inform a deceased patient's loved one of the death of their spouse or relative is the most difficult part of the process. You would think it gets easier but it's like the first time every time.

After conveying the sad news, people often react in bizarre ways, as if what has actually happened doesn't immediately sink in. I've heard responses such as the following: 'Who's going to feed the budgie now?' and 'He was going to mow the lawn today; I can't do it because of my arthritis. Would you be able to do it before you leave?' It's usually a short time later, often after the funeral has taken place, that the reality finally kicks in and the real grieving begins.

Tom and Jim had by now begun the journey to the hospital mortuary, while Carol and I gave our condolences to Rob's wife and left her with other members of her family who had since arrived at the house and were understandably upset. We had planned to meet Tom at the hospital, along with the fire service personnel who had kindly offered to assist us in the removal of Rob's body from the ambulance to the mortuary, and return the stretcher still in the back of our ambulance. So a short time after they'd arrived, and with the fire service also by now present, we met Tom at the hospital to assist him but discovered yet more problems had arisen.

At the time, only two mortuary drawers large enough to accommodate a bariatric patient like Rob were available... and they both had residents! Tom had nowhere to remove Rob's deceased body to, and therefore had to keep him contained on the floor in the back of his ambulance until the necessary arrangements could be made. With no immediate plan in sight, Carol and I took Tom's stretcher back to the ambulance station, and the fire service returned to their base too.

What occurred from that point on that day, and took up almost the rest of Tom and Jim's twelve-hour shift, was extremely degrading for Rob. He was left on the floor of the ambulance for several hours and eventually conveyed to another hospital approximately eight miles away. According to Tom, Rob's by now rigor mortised body was 'removed' from the ambulance in the same undignified way once again, and a post-mortem examination was carried out almost immediately upon their arrival. Performing a post-mortem examination on the same day as death is not the norm, but for some unknown reason it was deemed absolutely necessary in Rob's case. Perhaps it had something to do with his weight, or a lack of bariatric mortuary drawers at the time of his death. I've no idea.

Since attending to Rob, I have experienced similar predicaments involving bariatric patients who required admission to hospital in a timely manner, but where my crewmate and I were unable to remove them promptly due to their weight. Consequently, the patients deteriorated further on scene. Some we managed to keep alive and, following further assistance, rushed them to hospital in the nick of time. Others have died.

What the future holds for ambulance personnel, in terms of attending to bariatric patients, I can only surmise, but like I said earlier, the need to attend to obese patients is becoming progressively more frequent. Therefore, I envisage that to accommodate the ever expanding size of those within our modern day society, the number of bariatric mortuary drawers will be increased over the coming years, in addition to bariatric type ambulances replacing the present fleet type, and that these will be used to attend to every treble-nine or treble-one call, regardless of patients' age or weight. Watch this space!

Chapter 4
A Duty of Care

The 2006–2012 edition of the *JRCALC Guidelines* (a paramedics' bible) states that a duty of care *may* be defined as: 'The absolute responsibility of a healthcare professional to treat and care for a patient with a reasonable degree of skill and care'.

Every time an ambulance crew arrives at a patient's side, they automatically, from the outset, have a duty of care towards the patient or patients. That doesn't mean they *have to take* the patient to hospital, especially if the patient *doesn't want* to go to hospital and has the mental capacity to make that decision – determining mental capacity is a minefield that I won't attempt to explain here. If an ambulance crew forced a patient, who is fully conscious and who *has* the mental capacity, into the ambulance and conveyed them to hospital against their will, they could find criminal charges being brought against them and be struck off the professional register, and ultimately lose their jobs. Conversely, if a patient *doesn't want* to attend hospital but *does not* possess the mental capacity to make that decision, and could come to harm or could harm others, then a crew can 'legally' take particular actions to ensure that the patient is taken to a place of safety. That might be to A&E or, if lack of capacity is due to mental health – and there are no other medical illnesses or injuries present – an alternative and appropriate hospital or department.

If a Good Samaritan calls treble-nine for an ambulance because they've stumbled upon a drunken man laying in the gutter, and upon the crew arriving at the drunk's side he tells them to 'f**k off' – better known to ambulance personnel as Foxtrot Oscar

(FO), pertaining to the phonetic alphabet – then they cannot simply do as he asks. They can, however, temporarily 'stand-off' a safe distance from the abusive patient until the police arrive. But if the crew were to leave the patient and, subsequently, the drunk became unconscious and vomited, or worse still, choked on his own vomit and was later found dead in the gutter, the coroner would want answers. The circumstances surrounding the patient's death would be traced back to the attending crew who left him, and I don't think the coroner would settle for, 'Well he told me to f**k off sir, so why should I stick around and take that from the cheeky little scrote!?'

On the face of it, it's very easy to judge someone who is found drunk by the roadside. Paramedics *should* take in to account that the drunken man/woman may not be simply drunk. For instance, if a heart attack or stroke was imminent, yet unbeknown to the patient, then natural physiology isn't going to delay their mortality just because they're inebriated, is it? Who's to say a drunken person hasn't taken a suicidal cocktail of opiate-based prescription drugs as well as downed a bottle of whiskey?

We're really in no position to judge whether a drunken person warrants professional patient care and treatment or not, even if they tell you to f**k off. There may be mental health issues involved. They may have a head injury and be cerebrally irritated, or be suffering with low blood sugar levels – diabetic or not, we're all capable of having low blood sugar levels, especially after alcohol. Have you ever wondered why you're so hungry after an alcohol-fuelled night out on the town? That's because alcohol initially raises your blood sugar level, which stimulates the release of insulin to control the amount of sugar in your blood. When you have ceased drinking, your brain senses a reduction in sugar consumption, thus causing a hunger pang resulting in you being more than willing to eat a scabby horse if absolutely necessary!

So, who are we to assume that a less than polite drunken man or woman on the street is not simply hungry and experiencing one or two of the many side effects of low blood sugar levels, i.e. being irritable and aggressive? Of course, that's me looking at such a scenario from a broad perspective, but my point is that we have to accept that a drunken patient's behaviour, whether abusive or not, is not necessarily due to alcohol and that there may be another underlying condition, until proven otherwise. There are, without a doubt, thousands, maybe hundreds of thousands of people around the UK who would disagree with me and simply say a drunk is a drunk and a time waster. A lot are, yes, but it only takes a paramedic to misdiagnose one and they may find themselves struck off the professional register for failing to provide a duty of care, and also failing to act in the patient's best interests.

Unfortunately, ambulance personnel are frequently told to f**k off, and much worse. I've been called things that I won't write or even provide censored here. I don't take it personally though; they don't know me, so who cares what they think of me. I've regularly been called all the names under the sun by a drunken patient, before being informed that they're going to complain about me to the ambulance service for wanting to help them. It sounds ridiculous, doesn't it, but it does happen. Yes, it can get annoying, and yes you do sometimes feel like doing as they ask and Foxtrot Oscar.

During the earlier part of my career, when I was a rookie

ambulance technician, I allowed myself to be influenced by one or two unprofessional ambulance personnel, who educated me with their opinionated, cathartic rants about their perception of the general public, particularly how to deal with those under the influence of alcohol. However, as I've grown with experience, wisdom and knowledge and now possess a greater understanding of what was expected of me when I was granted professional registration by the Health and Care Professions Council, I no longer allow anyone to influence the way I assess or treat any class or type of patient, including drunks. By treating *all* patients with the same respect that I would like my own loved ones to receive, I leave nobody any ammunition to use against me if they decide to complain… not without having to lie in their letters of complaint, anyway. Instead, I approach each situation with tact, patience, compassion, understanding and CARE – that is, Cover Arse, Remain Employed. I'm only joking; one of my biggest pet-hates in the medical profession is clinicians who do things just to cover their arse in order to prevent a complaint. If you *act in the best interests of the patient* every time, and you can justify all of your actions, then you automatically cover your arse anyway, simple… you would think!

I'm afraid that's not so. Oh no. Even when you do act in the best interests of the patient, complaints still rear their ugly heads. I myself have had two written complaints made against me during my NHS career to date. I'll share those complaints with you here. I really don't mind, because I'm not ashamed to have received either of them; I'll let you decide whether I should be or not, and I'm happy to accept the fact that people's opinions do vary.

The first complaint made against me was from a patient's mother, who was also present while I was on scene at the pregnant teenager's address. A GP had arranged for an 'emergency' ambulance to convey her to the obstetrics unit because... wait for it... she had a cyst on her vagina. 'What!' I hear you shout. Yes, the patient, who was in the second trimester of pregnancy, informed me that she had told the doctor that she was happy to wait for her auntie to take her to hospital, but she would have to wait a couple of hours for her to arrive. The doctor had apparently insisted on an ambulance and therefore arranged one. Why? I don't know. She then reiterated to me that she was happy to wait for her auntie.

'That's fine,' I said, because unlike apples, ambulances and ambulance crew do not grow on trees. There is simply not enough government funding to put a sufficient number of them on the road as it is, without being used for conveying a patient to hospital because they have a cyst on their vagina. Good grief!

Patients, or their chaperone, would often ask me how many ambulances were operational at any given time per region of the county of Cheshire and Merseyside. That took a little extensive thinking to reckon up, so instead I would ask them to have a guess at how many they thought were available for one town with a population of approximately 65,000. Fifteen to twenty was the answer I was often given. When I informed them that the number of ambulances that were operational for one town with a population of 65,000 was in fact two, maybe three, they were astonished.

With the above in mind, and thinking 'yes, she needs an expert opinion on the cyst but not conveying by an emergency ambulance', I explained to the patient and her mother that, regardless of the GP arranging an ambulance, I was happy for them to wait for a lift from her auntie. I kept to myself the thought that my crewmate and I would be available for someone who *really* needs an ambulance; by that I mean available for someone experiencing crushing-like chest pain or severe difficulty in breathing. Or for someone in cardiac arrest; maybe even a child who had been knocked down by a car. Or a full-term expectant mother experiencing contractions two minutes apart, who may deliver at home with no pain relief or midwife to assist her or resuscitate the newborn if necessary. You know… *real* emergencies.

The patient's mother insisted that *we* take her daughter to hospital as the GP had arranged. I *politely* informed her that we would be no different than a taxi, and that I'd simply sit her daughter in a seat in the saloon of the ambulance, strap her in and she would be conveyed to hospital. Anyway, she insisted, so we took her!

Several weeks later, I was hauled into the office and handed a letter of complaint – complaints take time to get through the system. The complaint stated that I'd had a bad attitude towards their use of an ambulance, and that I had said to the patient's mother, using an abrupt tone, 'We're not a taxi service you know!' I was therefore asked to write a statement outlining my version of events, so I did. Included in that statement was a sentence with words to the effect of: 'There is a large adhesive transfer that appears prominently on the outside of the rear doors of the ambulance for all and sundry to clearly see, that states *This Is Not a Taxi. Use It, Don't Abuse It!'*

In that particular case, not only was the patient – or more so the patient's mother – abusing the ambulance service, but the GP was too. I was reprimanded for actually having the work ethic and desire to want to be available for somebody that might *really* need an emergency ambulance, but instead would potentially have to wait for a vehicle to arrive from further afield, possibly to the detriment of their life! What's the point in displaying a poster emphasising a message to not abuse the ambulance service, if the ambulance service condones the abuse of its resources? It's madness!

The second complaint actually came from an A&E consultant, who had received a completely different version of events from the patient that I'd attended to and treated. Allow me to explain.

My crewmate and I attended to a middle-aged lady who had slipped down the last three steps of her stairs and had landed awkwardly. She was screaming in absolute agony, still in the position she had landed, so I initially offered her the Entonox to self-administer while I ascertained some pertinent history. She didn't like the Entonox and so refused it after just several inhalations. Due to what I could see was a deformed lower left leg, I treated her for a closed fractured tibia and fibula, which was later confirmed by an x-ray in the A&E department. I explained to her that I could reduce or remove her pain by administering morphine.

'Morphine makes me sick,' she said.

'Do you have a genuine allergy to morphine or does it just make you sick?' I asked.

'Just sick,' she replied, still in agonising pain.

'I understand, but it makes a lot of people sick; it's one of the potential side effects of morphine,' I politely informed her. I also explained to her that, prior to me administering morphine, I could administer an anti-sickness drug – metoclopramide.

I asked her did she think that the excruciating pain she was experiencing was much worse than vomiting, or vice-versa. Her answer was that the pain was much worse, so she verbally consented to receiving both metoclopramide and morphine, and also signed my paperwork to state that she had given informed written consent. So after a set of observations and obtaining IV access, I administered the anti-sickness drug, while my crewmate prepared the morphine. Aware that morphine made her sick, I administered a small dose and awaited any adverse response from the patient, i.e. vomiting.

After several minutes of waiting, it became clear that she was fine, and so, with her verbal consent, I gave her a little more and once again waited: still no adverse response. 'Excellent,' I thought. After two small doses of morphine, the pain had reduced to a five out of ten. That enabled us to immobilise her deformed leg, assist her onto the stretcher and get her into the ambulance. There, we undertook secondary observations and then conveyed her to hospital.

Several weeks later, I was again hauled into the office and presented with a letter of complaint to read. That word-processed letter had a bold title headed, **'Inappropriate Administration of Morphine'**.

'Inappropriate!' I said. 'The woman was screaming in absolute agony with a suspected fractured leg. And she consented to it!' So, for the second time, I had to write a statement explaining my version of events. Prior to doing so, I asked for a photocopy of my patient report form.

Interestingly, there's a saying in the medical profession: *'If you didn't document it, you didn't do it'*. A solicitor would always find something to scrutinise you on, especially when their client has a financial motive, so I always pay close attention to that saying whenever I complete my patient clinical records, and that left me entirely confident to point out to the station manager that the patient had given me both verbal and written consent. I was also elated to be able to point out, because I had documented it, that the patient had not only consented to receiving morphine and all other drugs and treatment, but also that she had told me, following questioning and after doubly confirming with her husband, that she had *No Known Medicine Allergies*, which was recorded (as NKMA) on my documentation. In addition to that, I'd also recorded that I'd offered her a further dose of morphine but that she had declined it, and I was therefore unable to reduce her pain below a five out of ten, even though my empathetic intention was to reduce it to a zero. Furthermore, the patient had no symptoms of nausea and had not vomited throughout the entire time while in my care, including the journey to hospital. That too was recorded.

The letter of complaint stated that, a couple of hours after I'd admitted her to A&E, the patient had several bouts of severe vomiting. It became apparent that she'd told the A&E consultant that while she was in my care in her house, she'd informed me that she was allergic to morphine and could not have it in any form, but that I gave it to her anyway, against her will. That inaccurate statement... no, blatant lie, prompted the consultant to write to the ambulance service and complain about me, stating that I'd inappropriately administered morphine to a patient who was allergic to it.

Evidently, the A&E consultant hadn't bothered to read my

documentation. If she had taken the time to then she wouldn't have had any grounds to complain about my treatment of that patient. All I had done was provide a duty of care and act in the patient's best interests, and did my utmost best to alleviate the excruciating pain that she was experiencing, in addition to minimising the chance of her experiencing nausea and vomiting. In some respects, you can see why people tell me my job is a thankless one; though I'm still compelled to disagree.

No further actions were taken against me on either of the occasions explained above, because during the first incident I'd not 'had an attitude' and my crewmate, who I was working with at the time, backed me up on that. And, being caring and compassionate, I simply wanted to be available for an emergency. With regards to the second incident, my documentation was thorough and so everything I'd done, I had documented. Plus, the patient had given me verbal and written consent, which had been witnessed by my crewmate and the patient's husband. Anyway, I hold no grudges against either of the complainants, because I know the truth and that's all that matters to me. Fortunately, they're the only complaints I've had and I hope to keep it that way, though you can't please every patient, no matter how much care and compassion you show, so I'm sure another will come along one day.

This next incident has nothing to do with receiving a complaint, but it emphasises the term 'duty of care', and the importance of acting in the best interests of the patient at all times, regardless of a patient's incompliance or behaviour. And in this case, the patient became patients!

I was working solo on an RRV one spring day, and at 13:05 hours I was dispatched to attend to a thirty-three year old female experiencing shortness of breath. The dispatcher also informed me that there was no crew available to back me up, so I was to let them know on my arrival whether an ambulance was required or not. The patient had been able to make the treble-nine call herself, which in most cases, not all, is a good sign that their condition is not immediately life-threatening. Shortness of breath in a thirty-three year old could be one of a myriad of conditions, such as a heart attack, asthma or anxiety attack, chest infection, or pulmonary embolism – a clot in the lungs, which can be fatal – to name but a few. So I made my way to the address given, using blue lights and sirens, and arrived on scene within five minutes of being dispatched.

Vacating the RRV, I took the appropriate equipment into the house and there I was met by a lady pacing up and down the lounge. She was acting very anxious and breathing very fast and shallow. My first thought was, 'She's not experiencing shortness of breath due to a serious underlying problem, that's for sure.' She appeared very well perfused – that is, she had a nice pink colour due to an adequate amount of oxygen circulating her body. Her mannerisms and body language suggested that her shortness of breath was caused by a panic attack, but I had yet to find out why. For all I knew, it could have been due to a horrific recent or previous traumatic experience; approaching her like a bull in a china shop could have proved counter-productive.

Panic attacks – or hyperventilating, to be more precise – are one of the many run-of-the-mill emergencies frontline ambulance staff attend to. The root cause of a panic attack usually occurs from a personal and/or psychological source. For example stress, which can obviously be caused by an abundance of factors such as financial worries, post-traumatic stress disorder

(PTSD), relationship problems or fear of an upcoming event, such as an exam or job interview. The usual side effects of a panic attack are pins and needles down the arms and hands; also chest tightness, palpitations, and what is known as carpo-pedal spasm. This is when the wrist, and sometimes the feet, flexes and the fingers or toes gradually point inwards towards the body. All of the above mentioned side effects are caused by exhaling too much of the respiratory gas – carbon dioxide – due to rapid, shallow breathing.

My patient, whose name I didn't know at this point, continued to pace up and down the lounge rubbing her forehead, massaging the back of her neck and brushing her hands through her hair. She was extremely agitated. My assessment began with a global overview of the situation. My priority was to determine if she was likely to be violent or potentially unsafe towards me, herself or anybody else that may be in the house but not yet present in the lounge. In the absence of obvious danger, my approach would be to assess the situation by observing the scene for information to assist me in the care of her. I'd look for signs of violence, evidence of substance abuse, general environmental conditions, and any clue that might indicate previously existing medical problems such as diabetes which, as previously mentioned, can cause a person to become irritable and aggressive if sugar levels are low. I would also have to observe her for overt behaviour, such as language, thought, mood, intellect, activity, and body language for posture and gestures.

With a split-second global overview of the environment mentally noted, I adopted an empathetic and tactful approach towards her and so began by introducing myself using a calm, reassuring tone of voice.

'Good afternoon, my name's Andy, I'm a paramedic. What's your name?' I said, placing the equipment onto the floor.

'G-Gill,' she answered.

'OK Gill, I'm here to help you. What's your concern today?' I asked.

'I c-can't breathe or c-cope, I can't cope any longer. Go-go away, f**k off,' she said in a distressed and stuttered tone, and pacing back and forth, rubbing her hands through her hair.

'OK Gill, come and have a seat here and try and calm down. I'm here to help you, OK,' I said as I sat myself down on the sofa, attempting to demonstrate that I was relaxed and had all the time in the world to help her. Gill ignored my request and continued to pace about the room in an extremely nervous manner, so I left her as she was for a moment, while I informed ambulance control that I didn't need an ambulance at that time. I would contact them after assessing my patient further and reaching a decision on the most appropriate care pathway.

I calmly continued to reassure her.

'Gill, please come and have a seat so I can talk to you, come on. You called treble-nine so you must have thought you needed help, mustn't you? I'm here to help you,' I said, trying to assure her that I understood her angst.

'I c-can't cope anymore, there's never anyone around to h-help me, and I'm sc-scared of bleeding,' she said, continuing to pace up and down the lounge and struggling to talk and breathe at the same time.

'What do you mean, you're scared of bleeding, Gill?'

'I'm just sc-scared of bleeding, I can't cope and I'm sc-scared of bleeding. Just leave me alone, p**s off.'

'OK Gill, listen to me. I can see you're anxious, and the fact that you're not coping is fine. You're not the first person not to cope through life, and you won't be the last, I assure you. I can help you though, if you're not coping, but you do need to calm down, so please sit down and tell me why you're not coping, OK?'

'I c-can't keep still, I can't cope, I've had enough. I wanna go out, but what if I bl-bleed again?'

'Gill, come and sit down and take nice deep breaths. Then you can explain to me what your problems are.'

'I've had enough, I nee-need some h-help,' Gill stated, still breathing shallow, evidently in a confused state.

After a further fifteen minutes of reasoning with Gill, she finally sat down next to me on the sofa. With some respiratory coaching, she took long, deep breaths and her breathing gradually returned to a normal resting rate, but she remained fidgety, with a timid and nervous disposition. With Gill now a lot calmer I said,

'Right Gill, in your own time, explain to me what it is you're not coping with, and explain to me what you mean about being scared of bleeding. In your own time OK, there's no rush.'

As far as I was concerned, this call, which had been initially passed to me as a treble-nine, was not a life-threatening emergency at all, but a behavioural, social and welfare one that required understanding, tact and the utmost professionalism from me. A behavioural emergency implies a behaviour pattern that is presenting a threat to the well-being or life of the person exhibiting the behaviour. Such behaviour may also present a threat to the well-being or life of another. The dilemma with behavioural emergencies is to define 'normal' behaviour. There is no real definition of what normal is, or even what it means.

Have you ever been walking along the high street and thought he or she's a bit weird? I have, regularly, but that is just my opinion or perception of those people. Some people might look at me in the street and think the same about me. So what is normal behaviour? Ideas of normal vary by culture/ethnic group and family norms. The concept of abnormal behaviour implies behaviour that deviates from society's norms and expectations. That's a minefield to discuss, so I'm reluctant to go any further on the subject.

I was anticipating that I was going to be on scene with Gill for some time, and I was more than prepared to spend the rest of my shift on scene – just under seven hours – and beyond if absolutely necessary, to ensure that Gill's present predicament concluded with the help that she needed. She continued to act nervous, but nevertheless was able to explain to me a little about her history. She informed me that she had given birth to her first baby four weeks previous – I'd ascertained that the baby was asleep upstairs in a Moses basket. However, a short time after the birth of her daughter, she experienced a heavy vaginal bleed while out in public, which understandably caused her sheer embarrassment, and subsequently a fear of it happening again if she went out of the house. Following the vaginal bleed, she had an emergency gynaecological operation and had since been discharged from hospital, but wasn't coping with motherhood on her own.

By 'on her own' she meant the father of the baby, Gill's husband, had walked out on her while she was pregnant and she'd had no contact with him, and so nor had he with the baby. She also explained that assistance from family was limited. As a result, and having to look after the newborn baby and stay in all day through fear of another vaginal bleed, she often became anxious and hyperventilated. I allowed Gill to explain in detail what her concerns were, barely interrupting to ask her a question. I believed she simply needed someone to talk to and had wanted to for some time, and I was the only 'someone' at that time.

I'd been on scene, listening to Gill, for an hour or so and she had become a little more relaxed and open. She had explained to me about not being able to cope, what her operation had involved, her personal circumstances – which I've chosen not to include in full here – all of which couldn't have made life easy for Gill. It's quite intriguing for ambulance personnel how a patient who has never met you before feels able to open up because you're dressed in a green ambulance uniform. Would that happen out of uniform if you walked into someone's house and said, 'I'm an off-duty paramedic, air your dirty laundry to me'? I think they'd be on to the police in a flash; I know I would be. That is one of the many reasons why being a paramedic is often very interesting and occasionally very rewarding. The *majority* of the public trust us not to be judgemental towards them, and to treat them as an individual and with the utmost respect, which *most* ambulance personnel do, on a day-to-day basis.

After a long listening session, it had all become a lot clearer and so, even with my limited knowledge, I had made a provisional diagnosis. I had good reason to suspect that Gill was suffering from a condition called Post-Natal Depression (PND).

PND is a type of depression some women experience after

they've had a baby, not necessarily their first baby either. It usually develops in the first two months after childbirth, although in some cases it may not develop for some months after giving birth. There are several symptoms of post-natal depression, such as low mood, lethargy, feeling unable to cope and difficulty sleeping, to name but a few. But many women aren't aware that they even have the condition. It's quite normal to experience mood changes, irritability and tearfulness shortly after giving birth, but these normally disappear within a few weeks. However, if these symptoms persist, it could well be the result of post-natal depression.

The cause of post-natal depression is thought to be due to a combination of many things, rather than a single cause. These may include: the physical and emotional stress of looking after a newborn baby, individual social circumstances such as financial worries, lack of support from family, or even relationship problems. And in my opinion, PND, like *all* mental health problems, is often misunderstood, not only by the person suffering it but their spouse, relatives and, unfortunately, society in general. Only after help is sought by the sufferer, and the spouse and/or relatives are educated about their loved one's condition, does it become easier. Unfortunately, the majority in society still have a lot to learn about mental health; believe me, mental health problems are more common than you would think.

Throughout my career to date, I have attended to numerous individuals who have attempted suicide or repeatedly self-harmed by lacerating parts of their body and/or stubbing lit cigarettes out on themselves. Both of those disturbing acts of self-harm leave unsightly scars for life. I've even known a teenaged girl who was so mentally unwell that she forced a live hamster inside her vagina, breaking its neck as a consequence. And if that's not disturbing enough, she then forced two or three double 'A' batteries in there too. Some of you may laugh, but it's actually very, very sad that mental health problems cause such painful and bizarre behaviour. As a paramedic, I barely received any training on how to approach a patient with a mental health illness. I've had to learn through self-study, and by attending to patients with a range of mental health issues and learning from those experiences, occasionally researching particular conditions post-incident.

Anyway, with a provisional diagnosis noted, I had to consider the most appropriate care pathway for Gill's condition. While pondering over the options available to offer her, it occurred to me that I hadn't yet seen or heard the baby, because she had been asleep upstairs. So I began ascertaining further information from Gill, and also asked her if I could take some baseline observations, such as a pulse, SP02, blood pressure, blood glucose and temperature. Gill agreed. While undertaking those observations, I asked,

'Gill, what's your baby's name?'

'Jade,' she replied, more relaxed but still a little nervous.

'OK, when I've finished taking some obs, would you like to bring her down? I'd love to see her,' I said with motive. I wanted to check Jade over too, only visually; I didn't want to undertake any blood pressure or SP02 measurements on her, unless deemed absolutely necessary. The reason I wanted to see Jade was to confirm that my initial diagnosis of PND hadn't caused Gill to intentionally or unintentionally harm her newborn – physically or neglectfully.

Gill quite calmly went upstairs to get Jade. A minute or so later, she came back into the lounge and sat down again, with Jade fast asleep in her arms. I glanced at her daughter, who was dressed in a baby-grow which appeared clean, as did her face and hands. Although I hadn't thoroughly checked Jade over, I was satisfied so far and therefore continued to talk through some options with Gill for her to consider, in order to help her. They centred on me potentially contacting her GP and requesting him to visit Gill at home – it was unlikely that she would have had the confidence to leave the house, based on what she had previously told me. By having her GP visit, I had hoped that he would assess her and potentially prescribe some anti-depressants at the very least.

I also considered contacting Gill's husband, who she had separated from, and also close family members, and ask them to come to the house while Gill was in my care. If they came over, I could discuss Gill's health and welfare with them, face to face, and hopefully leave the scene with peace of mind, having discussed and agreed on a plan of action with them. A short period went by and discussions seemed to be going well with Gill, and I'd felt like I was getting close to arriving at a safe and appropriate care pathway and would soon be able to clear from the scene, then the process of Gill receiving professional help could have begun.

Unfortunately, progress was short-lived. While discussing options and with Jade in her arms, Gill unexpectedly, and to my alarm, became agitated again. She began tapping one heel on the floor and alternately raising and lowering one thigh really quickly, as if she had too much pent-up energy and was trying to use some of it up with rapid limb movements. When the leg movements stopped, she began rocking back and forth, and it wasn't to get Jade off to sleep; she was already fast asleep. At the time, I didn't know why she was doing that, but I'm now led to believe it was a form of self-soothing. So with Jade's safety in mind, I offered my assistance.

'Gill, do you want me to hold her for a bit? I've got children too, so I know how to hold babies,' I said, trying to help.

'No, no, it's OK,' she said as she abruptly stood. 'I'll put her down.'

I acknowledged Gill's refusal and thought she was going to place Jade onto the soft cotton sofa opposite us, so I glanced away for a few seconds. When I turned back around, Gill had actually placed Jade on her back along the edge of a dining table. I'm sure my heart momentarily stopped! I leapt to my feet, at what felt like a hundred miles per hour, and hurtled towards the table.

'Gill, Gill, let me take hold of Jade, you go and bring the Moses basket down, OK, we'll pop her back in there so she can sleep comfortably. The table's not very comfortable, is it?' I said calmly, trying to hide the sudden burst of adrenaline that had been released. Gill frowned at me, with a look of confusion on her face, and then handed Jade over to me. She then left the room and went back upstairs.

I was relieved that Jade was safely in my arms. However, in order to *act in the best interests of the patient/s*, I had no choice but to forget the options we had discussed and escalate my concerns further. I couldn't be sure whether Gill was suffering with PND in isolation, or whether she had a more serious mental health condition that was outside my scope of clinical knowledge to diagnose. The predicament had worsened, because what had started out as one patient had now become two. I not only had to ensure Gill received the appropriate help and support, but also that Jade would be safe and well too.

My mind began to race a little and I started to ask myself some very uncomfortable questions: 'Why had she put Jade on the edge of a table, potentially causing serious, maybe even fatal harm had she fallen off? Should I contact social services? Should I ring Gill's husband and ask him to come to the house, regardless of the current marital status? Should I contact the mental health services and try to get her admitted? What if I had left after arranging for a GP to visit; I might not have witnessed what I just had.'

Gill came back down the stairs and into the lounge with the Moses basket. I asked her to sit back down. I put Jade into the Moses basket and then sat beside Gill once again.

'Gill, we need to discuss further what we're going to do today, OK?' I said, still a little shaken from what I'd witnessed. 'I think a visit to the hospital might do you some good, give you some rest. I can contact your husband or mum, if you wish, and let them know. What do you think?'

'No, I don't need hospital, I'm fine,' she said, frowning, staring at the floor and rocking back and forth.

'Gill, you're not coping very well are you? You said it yourself earlier that you needed help, so why don't you let me arrange for an ambulance to take you to hospital for some checks, hey? I'm sure your husband can come home and look after Jade for a bit, can't he?' I said, attempting to gently persuade her.

'No, I'm fine, really, I don't need hospital.'

'OK Gill, why were you going to leave Jade on the table?' I reluctantly asked.

'Cause I can't cope… it's hard, I just can't cope,' she said, frowning and rubbing her hands through her hair.

'Well if you can't cope, let's get you to hospital and see what they can do for you,' I said, hoping for a nod of agreement. Gill directed her eyes towards Jade in the Moses basket.

'She drives me crazy, screamin' all the time. This is the quietest she's been in four weeks. I won't cope when she wakes up. I feel like killin' her.'

That last comment made my heart sink and my stomach churn. Did she literally mean that or did she mean it as a generalised figure of speech, as occasionally we all do? I continued to question Gill, and at the same time tried to reassure her.

That questioning and reassurance continued for a further hour. During that hour I'd contacted ambulance control to update them on how I was and why I'd been on scene for so long. And in that time, Gill had also repeated comments similar to what she had said earlier, about killing her baby. A further thirty minutes passed by and I'd continued to try to persuade Gill to attend hospital, and also tried to make further attempts to contact her mum and husband on the telephone, but to no avail. After a further several attempts, Gill's mum answered. I discreetly explained the situation to her and why I was at Gill's address. She was obviously keen to get to Gill and Jade as quickly as possible. While waiting for her to arrive, I continued encouraging Gill to attend hospital; but I wasn't thinking A&E department, rather a direct referral to a mental health hospital for an immediate mental health assessment.

Just a short time prior to her mum arriving, Gill and I reached a compromise: She agreed to go direct to the mental health hospital, as long as Jade could go with her. I settled for that decision but had to make a few phone calls in order to arrange it, as it was unusual for a patient to be able to take their child into hospital with them, especially when a referral for a mental health assessment had been made. Nevertheless, after I'd explained to the doctor the history of events that had unfolded that afternoon, Gill's request was granted.

I was relieved that she had finally agreed, after she'd continually insisted that she didn't need to attend hospital. Had we not reached a compromise, I would have had no choice but to consider alternative options, such as requesting the police to attend the scene and section her under section 136 of the Mental Health Act, which would have resulted in her being taken to a place of safety – most likely the A&E department – until her mental health could be assessed. The process of sectioning her wouldn't have been straightforward however, as section 136 can only be executed in a public place. The patient cannot be detained under section 136 while in their own home, and so the only way it could have been done would have been to persuade Gill to step outside of her front door and then detain her. That sounds awful, doesn't it? But that often occurs, for the patient's own safety and the safety of others too.

By the time Gill's mum arrived at the house, I'd been on scene for nearly four hours with Gill and was beginning to feel mentally exhausted. The ambulance that I'd arranged to take Gill and Jade to hospital arrived on scene, and so Gill, with less reluctance than I had anticipated, walked out of the front door. The crew secured them both with safety straps and conveyed them safely to hospital. I saw out the remainder of my shift and went home. Throughout that evening, I couldn't help but ponder over the incident and kept wondering what the outcome for Gill and Jade would be.

The following day, while on duty once again, I decided to follow-up Gill and Jade's welfare by personally visiting the relevant health care professionals that had cared for them. What I learnt saddened me. Gill had been mentally assessed and unfortunately sectioned under the Mental Health Act. I could only assume that following professional assessment, Gill had been diagnosed with more than post-natal depression and was deemed to be a threat to herself and possibly Jade, too. According to the nurse, Gill's husband wasn't interested in taking responsibility for Jade. Fortunately though, Jade was able to stay with her grandmother while Gill remained in hospital.

Although it was very sad to hear that Gill was not suffering PND in isolation, and that Jade had been taken away from Gill as a consequence, I stood by my decision to escalate the incident further, though it had been an extremely difficult decision to make at the time. I had acted in the best interest of both Gill and Jade and had therefore provided a duty of care to them both. As a consequence, Gill would be appropriately treated and Jade would come to no harm. Having said that, I really didn't believe that Gill had wanted to harm Jade; I believed it was the effects of her mental health at the time that caused her to be unaware of the danger she had placed Jade in when she laid her on the table. And I didn't believe she genuinely wanted to kill her. Then again, mental health problems can cause people to commit the most peculiar acts of behaviour without a moment's notice; often without even realising they're acting the way they are. I've attended to countless mentally ill patients throughout my career, and I assure you it's very disturbing and very sad to experience.

Whether Jade was ever returned to her mum I never did find out, and unfortunately a severe mental illness often involves a long road to recovery. Sadly, some patients are never deemed mentally stable enough to be alone around their children ever again.

The Dark Side

Chapter 5
Stairwell of Hell

Like many paramedics, when I get ready for work I do so with the intention of appearing as an ambassador for the NHS ambulance service; a registered paramedic who is there to symbolise the profession for what it stands for, and to help those sick and injured patients in need of a high standard of care. Some of us like to adopt the attitude that if we give the patient the impression that we are able to look after ourselves, then the patient will perceive us as able to look after them, too.

We prepare a clean, green coloured uniform in advance – green is supposedly a calming colour – pressing the shirt so the creases appear likely to lacerate the fingers of anyone who dares glide their hand along the length of a single sleeve. We polish our boots so they shine so bright that a drill sergeant from the elite regiment, the *Grenadier Guards*, would be proud to wear them. OK, maybe not *that* good! We have a clean, close shave (even some of the women) and a hot shower, and ensure that our finger nails are short so bacteria are unable to breed under them. We also make sure that our hair is neat and tidy. Once dressed, we then clip our I.D. badge to the left-hand breast pocket, just under the UK Ambulance Services' crest – the sign of Asclepius, the Greek god of medicine and healing. We might also place our pen-torch and tuffcut scissors into the tailor-made, pen-sized pockets on the left-hand sleeve. Then we stand tall, with our shoulders back, and hope to appear to the public as smartly dressed, proud UK paramedics.

Of course, all that effort goes to rat shit when you respond to a road traffic collision (RTC) in the pouring rain and are presented with a car on its roof in a saturated field. Before you know it, you're kneeling in mud and your nice shiny boots are covered in sludge, and you're sweating profusely. If that wasn't enough, adrenaline pumps through your veins while you precariously squeeze through the smashed passenger window in order to check for a pulse in the unconscious occupant, who has blood seeping from their ears.

Alternatively, you're called to an address – before nine o'clock in the morning – which should have a warning sign on the front door that says: *'Take your shoes off, you'll get them filthy in here!'* There you find, surrounded by empty cans of high-strength lager, a dishevelled alcoholic, intoxicated, rolling around in his own urine and faeces, in addition to the remnants of vomit that have become a permanent feature on the sticky, uncarpeted lounge floor.

Consequently, I do sometimes ask myself why we make so much of an effort to look smart and professional for work. We might as well go on duty like forensic scientists at a crime scene, dressed in a white, all-in-one *Umper Lumper* suit, with the hood up and a white face mask to match. I'm sure that would make more sense.

That brings me to this next incident, which involved a very unfortunate young man who was diagnosed with epilepsy after sustaining a head injury from a horrific road traffic collision five years previous. It was 6:45 a.m. on a cold winter's morning and I'd just arrived at the ambulance station, fifteen minutes in advance of commencing a twelve-hour day shift. My uniform was fresh and crisp, having been meticulously pressed the night before. I was clean shaven and my boots were polished to a high standard. At 7 a.m., I'd be ready to take on another day.

No sooner had I arrived, I and my crewmate, Jess, were asked by the night crew to respond to a job for them as they were due to finish at 7 a.m. and understandably didn't want to finish late. That is one of the downsides of the job, getting a late treble-nine call, but if you're the only crew available then it's absolutely imperative to accept the call and respond without delay, if you want to remain on the professional register. In the UK, HCPC Professionally Registered Paramedics have been struck off the register for refusing to attend emergency calls just minutes before their shift was due to finish. Refusing an emergency call is an absolute no-no in the paramedical profession, because to refuse an emergency call rather contradicts the word 'Professional' in the title. It goes against one of the many standards of proficiency that health care professionals sign up to every two years; that is, as previously mentioned: *'To act in the patient's best interests at all times'.*

Anyway, I digress a little. Of course we weren't going to allow our colleagues to finish perhaps an hour and a half late for the sake of us having to start our shift fifteen minutes early. So without chance to even begin vehicle or equipment checks, we immediately threw our personal protective equipment on to the ambulance and proceeded to the address given.

The nature of the call passed to us was to attend to a twenty-four year old male, known epileptic, who was convulsing. Now, before I continue, allow me to explain a little about epilepsy.

There are over 40 types of epilepsy and over 200 types of seizure, and I have to confess I'm no expert when it comes to having much knowledge about epilepsy or seizures. What I can tell you is that if you have a seizure, it doesn't necessarily mean that you'll be diagnosed as having epilepsy. Seizures occur for many reasons, while epilepsy, on the other hand, is a diagnosed condition. To keep it simple for both you and me, I'll explain epilepsy like this: There is electrical activity happening within our brain all the time, and an epileptic seizure occurs when there is a sudden surge of intense electrical activity. Try to imagine a 'thunderstorm' in the brain – a brainstorm, if you like. This 'brainstorm' causes the messages in the brain to become mixed up. The intense electrical activity causes a temporary disturbance to the way the brain normally functions. The result is an epileptic seizure.

The cause of epilepsy in an individual isn't always clear. It could be because of brain damage caused by a difficult birth – the brain may have received an inadequate amount of oxygen for a significant period of time. It may be caused by a traumatic head injury, a stroke, or an infection of the brain such as meningitis, to name just several of an abundance of potential causes. All Jess and I knew was that the patient was a diagnosed epileptic, but having that information was in itself very helpful. Forewarned is forearmed, as they say.

Jess and I arrived and parked up close to the address. The location given to us was on the top floor of a four-storey block of flats on a rundown, poverty-stricken council estate. We vacated the cab, grabbed the appropriate equipment from the saloon and proceeded towards the building.

On arriving at the ground floor, and faced with the stairwell, I stopped and thought, 'Is it worth getting the carry-chair now, just in case he needs to go to hospital?' Often, known epileptics have ceased convulsing by the time the ambulance crew arrive and are usually in what is called a post-ictal state, which simply means they are no longer convulsing. Most epileptics control their condition very well with medication, and so they usually rouse to a state of full consciousness after a short period, while in the attending paramedic's presence. Many blatantly refuse to be taken to hospital, even if we advise them to go for further observations, and so a carry-chair is seldom required. Given that the patient was on the top floor, which would mean Jess and I having to ascend six sets of concrete steps – two sets per floor, each set having eight steps, a total of forty-eight – I decided it would be sensible to take the carry-chair straight in, just in case the patient was unwell enough to warrant a visit to A&E.

Jess hurried back to the ambulance for the chair, while I began lugging the equipment up the forty-eight concrete steps, scrunching my nose up along the way against the aroma of stale and fresh urine that wafted from each floor. Having reached the top floor and walked along the landing, I arrived outside the patient's flat. Jess had almost caught up with me and so followed a short distance behind. The door was closed but unlocked, so I let myself in and entered the small hallway.

'Hello, ambulance service!' I shouted. There was barely any room to manoeuvre with the door open before yet another flight of stairs was in front of me.

'Up here!' a female voice yelled.

Jess was by now right behind me, so we both proceeded up the stairs towards the voice. When I pushed what I assumed was once a white, but now a yellow-tinged, nicotine-stained lounge door open, what we found was a room that resembled something normally seen on ITV's *Grimefighters.* An offensive smell immediately hit our olfactory senses, causing mine and Jess's noses to scrunch up once again. The walls were black and yellow with filth and nicotine stain to match the door, and had evidently not been painted since the building's completion in 1972. The filthy, once beige coloured, carpeted floor was scattered with disordered clutter, dirty laundry, and crockery that hadn't been washed since food had been eaten off it several weeks previous, judging by the bits of mouldy leftovers embedded on it. There was a TV and a cabinet in the corner, which I assumed was once a glass cabinet – the glass had been smashed, possibly during a convulsion, who knows? The patient lay on a torn, brown leather sofa that had seen better days, violently convulsing.

The treble-nine caller was the patient's mum. She appeared anxious and upset. That was understandable, as she was witnessing her son's body in a state of rigid spasm. He was sweating profusely and his eye lids were flickering, and blood was dripping down his chin from biting down on his tongue; that is common during an epileptic seizure and meant I couldn't consider the use of an oral airway adjunct because his teeth were clenched. Jess and I quickly walked over to the patient and knelt down on the filth-ridden rug that had obviously seen better days too. A white, all-in-one *Umper Lumper* suit would have most certainly been handy on this occasion!

I began questioning his mum while, with the assistance of Jess, simultaneously started assessing and treating him.

'OK love, what's his name?' I asked, while reaching for a nasal airway adjunct from the paramedic bag.

'Daniel,' she replied, tearfully.

'And I believe Daniel is a diagnosed epileptic, is that right?' I asked, while applying KY jelly to the malleable plastic tube.

'Yeah, from a car crash five years ago.'

'Oh, right,' I replied, before saying to Jess, 'forget the sats and BP, just get me a blood glucose, and if it's normal, draw up two ampoules of diazemuls as quick as you can please, hun.' I would normally only ask for one ampoule – an ampoule is a sealed glass capsule containing a drug in liquid or powdered form – but I decided it would be a good idea to have more of the drug pre-prepared, as this would prevent any delay in administering it in the unusual event that I needed more while descending the stairwell.

While Jess pin-pricked Daniel's finger for a drop of blood, I continued questioning his distressed mum.

'How long has he been convulsing for, this morning?'

'I don't know. I rang him at quarter past six and he didn't answer, so I came over and let myself in and found him convulsing,' she replied, as I attempted to insert the adjunct into his right nostril, which is the most suitable nostril anatomically.

'And how long did it take you to get over here?' I asked, struggling to get the nasal adjunct suitably in place because of the anatomy of his crooked nose.

'About twenty-five minutes or so,' she answered, as I successfully inserted the adjunct into his left nostril instead.

'Has he not stopped convulsing since you've been here then?' I asked, applying an oxygen mask to his face and switching the cylinder to high flow.

'No, not at all,' she replied.

'When was his last seizure; does he normally control it well?' I asked, cutting the sleeve of his rugby shirt to locate a suitable vein for cannulation.

'He's not had a seizure for a while, must be six or twelve months, I think. He takes Epilim though, if that's any help.'

'OK, thank you. Right Jess, we need to get him to hospital ASAP,' I said. 'But first I need to try and stop him from convulsing, so we can lift him down the stairs and the outside stairwell,' I muttered.

What Daniel was suffering from was a life-threatening condition called status epilepticus. Yes, I know it sounds like the name of a slave-come-gladiator during the days of the Roman Empire, but it is a medical emergency that can kill if not brought under control in a timely manner. Status epilepticus *may* be defined as a continuous seizure lasting for at least 20-30 minutes, or two or more discrete seizures between which the patient does not regain consciousness. It is life-threatening because the longer a seizure lasts, the less likely it is to stop on its own or with emergency medicines, one of which I'd asked Jess to prepare for me – diazemuls.

Diazemuls is an anti-convulsant/skeletal muscle relaxant that contains diazepam. Paramedics carry diazepam in two forms, one as a milky coloured liquid for intravenous administration, and the second a clear liquid to be given rectally. Rectal diazepam is usually given to convulsing children, where appropriate, because cannulating a child can sometimes prove more difficult than adults. Occasionally, administering rectal diazepam to an adult may be the paramedic's only option, and as unpleasant as it is to administer it rectally to an adult, it can have the same desired effect on the patient as with IV administration.

I remember an incident not long after I'd qualified as a paramedic. My crewmate, an ambulance technician, and I were called to a residential home to attend to a fifty-odd year old man with learning difficulties. On our arrival, the patient had ceased convulsing, so I took the opportunity to cannulate while he was stationary. Being a rookie, I didn't think of securing the cannula with anything stronger than the usual adhesive dressing. Shortly after cannulating, the patient began convulsing again and subsequently knocked the cannula out. While he continued to convulse, I palpated for another vein in order to obtain a second IV cannula, but with no joy. The patient continued to violently convulse, so my crewmate and I had no choice but to pull down his trousers and underwear slightly and endure the sight and nauseating stench from his double incontinence, which commonly occurs during an epileptic seizure. I then had to squeeze rectal diazepam between his soiled butt cheeks, into his rectum – blimey, I'm not exactly selling the job to anyone here!

Fortunately though, the drug worked and he stopped convulsing. I learnt a valuable lesson during that incident and have never had to administer rectal diazepam since, with the exception of a four month old baby, but that was a piece of cake compared to the former. Whenever I attend to an epileptic, or any other patient whose condition may cause them to have a seizure, such as an unconscious diabetic with low blood sugar levels, I make sure that I secure the cannula with a net-like bandage, making it almost impossible to be pulled out by the patient.

Jess had pin-pricked Daniel's finger for a drop of blood and measured his blood glucose levels. They were normal, so I was happy that the cause of Daniel's convulsing wasn't due to life-threateningly low blood sugar levels. Obtaining a blood glucose measurement was imperative, as convulsing isn't dissimilar to isometric exercise. Isometric exercises are a type of strength training in which the joint angle and muscle length do not change during contraction. Isometrics are done in static positions, rather than being dynamic through a range of motion, so Daniel would be metabolising calories, or 'burning sugar', causing his blood sugar levels to drop too. Low blood sugar levels could have made Daniel's condition even more complicated to manage, and had they been low would have required me to infuse some glucose through his veins before considering epilepsy as a cause of his seizure, regardless of the fact that he was a diagnosed epileptic.

Jess began to prepare the diazemuls, but before I could administer the drug, I needed to obtain IV access. I gripped Daniel's wrist tightly, to avoid it sliding through my hand as he was dripping with sweat and I was beginning to as well. I applied a tourniquet to his right arm and chose a medium sized cannula from the paramedic bag, and waited for a viable vein to appear. After tapping his arm for thirty seconds or so, to my disappointment, no vein appeared. So I unclipped the tourniquet and applied it to his left arm. Again, I tapped away hoping for a vein to appear. There was nothing. Jess could see I was having difficulty, but continued to prepare the IV diazemuls in the event that I would shortly be successful in my efforts.

The thought of carrying Daniel down the stairs from the flat, still convulsing, was playing on my mind, and I'm sure it was on Jess's mind too. It would be fraught with danger. If there's one flight and the patient is conscious, it's not too bad... depending on the patient's weight, that is. I estimated Daniel to weigh about fourteen stone. Fourteen stone isn't too bad with a single flight of stairs, but when there's more than one flight of stairs to descend, as in this case, carrying a convulsing patient would be an absolute nightmare. So I had to get IV access or we'd be lifting a convulsing patient down the stairwell, or worse, Daniel could deteriorate in to a cardiac arrest while still in his flat; an absolute hellish nightmare for any ambulance crew.

Daniel had been convulsing for possibly thirty minutes prior to our arrival, and was still convulsing: He needed diazemuls, and fast! I had to make a decision: Administer rectal diazepam or cannulate another limb? In haste, I took the decision that I wasn't going to give up on obtaining IV access just yet. Instead, I took his socks off and applied the tourniquet to the ankle of his spasming right leg. I waited for a vein to appear. 'Come on, show yourself,' I thought, as Daniel continued to violently convulse. No joy. With sweat beginning to drip from my forehead, I removed the tourniquet and reapplied it to his left ankle. I tapped away at the top of the inside of the ankle but nothing appeared, initially. Then, a poor excuse for a blue tinge appeared and the vein began to slightly swell below the surface of the skin. 'Excellent! Here we go,' I thought.

'Jess, hold his leg as still as you can, I've only got one shot at this. If I miss, we're up shit creek without a paddle and we'll have to lift him all the way down, convulsing,' I said, anticipating hell if that was the case. Sweat continued to roll down my forehead and face, and I could feel my shirt sticking to my back and to the underneath of my arm pits. Jess took hold of Daniel's leg and held it as still as she could under the circumstances, while I lined up the sharp needle with the blue tinge near his ankle. With the cannula in my hand, and trying to keep in line with the vague, blue tinge, I pierced the skin. A flashback appeared in the chamber, so I advanced the needle further and then withdrew slightly and awaited a secondary flashback to appear along the length of the clear plastic tube. As it appeared, I unclipped the tourniquet, applied digital (thumb) pressure and then withdrew the needle completely, disposing of it safely. I screwed the Luer-Lock to the end and quickly secured it in place with an adhesive dressing and a net-like bandage, before flushing it with a pre-filled, ten-millilitre syringe of sodium chloride to confirm patent IV access.

Daniel was still convulsing and beginning to look progressively paler, even with supplemental oxygen being administered, and he was also wringing wet from the excessive sweat produced from what was, in effect, an intense exercise session. Jess passed me the syringe containing the milky-coloured contents. I opened up the injection port of the cannula and slowly squeezed the syringe, allowing a small amount of the drug to enter his veins, and waited for it to have a positive effect, i.e. for him to cease convulsing.

Daniel's mum looked on, obviously concerned for her son's life. I continued to inject further doses of diazemuls through the cannula, intermittently alternating my eyes between Daniel's spasming body and the amount of the drug disappearing from the syringe. Two milligrams had gone. Then four, six, eight, nine and in less than a minute, ten milligrams had gone. Daniel's convulsing gradually reduced and then stopped completely. Jess and I let out a deep sigh of relief.

Our work was not complete yet, though. As expected, Daniel remained in an unconscious state and we now had to get him from his flat into the ambulance. Pre-empting extraction from the flat, Jess prepared the carry-chair. Now that Daniel had stopped convulsing, it was imperative that we began the process of vacating the flat and descending the 'stairwell of hell' as fast as possible, as epileptics sometimes start convulsing again even after receiving diazemuls. Jess placed the carry-chair next to the sofa and, between the two of us, we top 'n' tailed Daniel onto the chair, leaving his nasal adjunct and oxygen mask in place. I placed a blanket around him for warmth and to prevent his arms from overhanging the sides. Next, he was secured in place with a strap around his upper body and one around his feet, to prevent him from kicking out in the event he began convulsing again.

Instructing Daniel's mum to follow, and asking her to kindly carry our equipment, we wheeled him out of the lounge and carefully lifted him down the first set of stairs and out of the front door. Pushing the chair along the outside landing, I kept observing Daniel for any obvious signs that he might start convulsing again, such as his arms shaking.

Now at the top of the steps, and with Daniel motionless and unconscious, Jess took hold of the lower end of the chair while I remained at the upper end.

'One-two-three lift,' I said to Jess. We began descending the first set of eight steps. Jess periodically looked over her shoulder to ensure she didn't misplace her footing and slip or fall backwards. We reached the bottom of the first set and so placed the chair down onto the ground for a very brief rest. Then Jess and I gave each other the nod to go for the next set. 'One-two-three lift.'

And so we began the descent. However, midway down, the chair suddenly felt somewhat more difficult to carry. Daniel's head hyperextended, that is, it jerked backwards into my stomach. He was having another seizure!

'Hold on tight, Jess, and keep lifting until we get to the bottom of this set,' I instructed. I had my sweaty fists tightly clenched around the handle of the chair, doing my utmost best not to let go. My own body went in to a rigid and tense state, and we were both sweating and panting with the sheer intensity and exhaustion brought about by lifting a convulsing body. It was becoming an exercise session for us too. When we reached the bottom of that set, we lowered the chair to the ground for another very brief rest and to administer a further dose of diazemuls.

I asked Daniel's mum, who was looking on with concern, to pass me the paramedic bag, then asked Jess to stand behind the carry-chair to prevent it from tipping backwards. Leaving the strap around his upper body, and with the chair secured by Jess's bodyweight, I grabbed the syringe containing the remaining ten milligrams of diazemuls and then rummaged around the blanket covering his feet. When a patient convulses while sat on the carry-chair, what can sometimes happen is they literally shake and slide down the chair, as if escaping from a strait-jacket, so before that occurred, I quickly located the cannula in his left foot, flicked the cap open and administered more diazemuls, slowly squeezing one, two, three milligrams through the injection port. Several seconds later, the convulsing ceased once more. We were now able to continue our descent.

'Right, are you ready?' I said to Jess. She gave a nod. So with the chair teetering over the edge, I said, 'One-two-three lift.' Off we went again, hoping that Daniel would remain in a post-ictal state for the duration of not only the lift down the remaining set of steps but en route to hospital, too.

We continued descending each set of eight steps, anticipating that Daniel might start convulsing again. Fortunately, to our relief, he didn't and we finally reached the ground floor level.

Beads of sweat continued to drip down our faces, and my shirt clung tightly to my body. We hurriedly manoeuvred the chair around the pathways towards the ambulance and got him on-board. There, we unstrapped him and carefully top 'n' tailed him onto the stretcher. He remained unconscious and still tolerated the tube inserted into his nose.

'Right, my love, take a seat for me and pop your seatbelt on,' I said to Daniel's distraught mum. 'Jess, get a sats, a blood pressure and a temp, while I put the three lead ECG on.' Conveyance to A&E with as little delay as possible was vital, but first I needed to see his heart rate and rhythm, following what had been the unknown but probably lengthy amount of time he'd been convulsing. Prolonged seizures can cause the heart to struggle considerably, enough to cause significant damage.

Jess undertook the observations I'd requested, which were all as expected following an epileptic seizure. His sats were ninety-six percent on oxygen. His blood pressure was 160mmHg systolic. He had a temperature of 38.5 centigrade. His high temperature may well have been the cause of his seizure; an infection can and often does cause epileptics to convulse, even if they control their condition adequately, or even if they've not had an episode for some considerable time.

Now wired up to the ECG, I monitored Daniel's heart rate and rhythm. It was pumping away at 137 BPM, which was normal following a prolonged episode of convulsing. Due to the amount of fluid he'd lost through convulsing and his high temperature, I decided to attach a drip to the cannula in Daniel's leg and open the pinch a little, to allow fluid to gradually hydrate him while in my care. The fluid therapy could then also be continued while he was in the A&E department.

Jess conveyed a pre-alert message to A&E resus, requesting an anaesthetist to be on standby. If Daniel began convulsing again, he may have needed anaesthetising and intubating to prevent him from deteriorating in to cardiac arrest or sustaining irreversible brain damage. With the pre-alert message conveyed, Jess mobilised to A&E under emergency conditions, but Daniel began to convulse again en route, despite having received thirteen milligrams of diazemuls so far. I had to administer a further three milligrams to once more cease his convulsing. That carried risks of his respiratory rate reducing. While in transit, and taking that risk in to account, I monitored his sats and the rise and fall of his chest for any compromise in his respiratory rate, in addition to further blood pressure measurements.

When we arrived at A&E, Jess opened up the rear doors, lowered the ramp and, with Daniel's mum following behind, we wheeled the stretcher inside the cubicle where the department staff were waiting, including the anaesthetist Jess had requested. While transferring Daniel over to the hospital bed, I gave my handover to the lead doctor.

'This is known epileptic, Daniel, twenty-four years old. Daniel was diagnosed with epilepsy five years ago following a head injury from a car crash.

'Daniel is on Epilim; last seizure was approx six to twelve months ago, according to his mum. His mum was unable to contact Daniel this morning, so she went to his flat and found him having a seizure. We're not sure how long he'd been convulsing for prior to our arrival, but it may have been thirty minutes or more.

'On our arrival, Daniel was convulsing, pale and sweating profusely. He's bitten down on his tongue, but airway remained clear and unobstructed. Unable to insert an oral airway adjunct due to clenched teeth, so a nasal airway was inserted and tolerated, and high flow oxygen administered.

'IV access routes poor, but I managed to secure a line in his lower left leg.

'Blood glucose normal, so with low blood sugar levels ruled out as a cause of his convulsing, I administered ten milligrams of diazemuls to good effect, and a further three milligrams administered while egressing from the location to the ambulance, as he started convulsing again.

'While en route, Daniel had a further seizure, so a further three milligrams was administered. He has not convulsed since and has remained unconscious.

'His initial blood pressure measurement was one hundred and sixty systolic and has remained similar en route. His heart rate has been fluctuating between one hundred and thirty and one hundred and forty-five BPM.

'Daniel's got a temperature of thirty-eight point five. Present infections unknown. Are there any questions?'

Daniel's mum looked on as the doctors and nurses immediately began to repeat all of the observations that Jess and I had undertaken, to compare and determine whether there were any signs of improvement or deterioration. Daniel remained unconscious but continued to breathe adequately by himself. However, not long after we'd transferred him onto the resus bed, he began to convulse yet again. Since our job was complete, we left Daniel in the expert hands of the doctors to treat him with alternative drugs that would hopefully bring his convulsing under control.

While the doctors battled with Daniel's condition, Jess and I went outside to allow the cold air to evaporate the sweat on our faces. We were both absolutely exhausted from the physical intensity of the incident. After a short recovery period, I completed my paperwork and signed out two ampoules of diazemuls from the drug safe, while Jess put all of the equipment back in its correct place in the ambulance. After twenty minutes, we were ready to clear with ambulance control, hoping we'd be sent back to station for a well-earned brew; well, carrying a fourteen stone patient down forty-eight steps is thirsty work, after all! And… it was only the *start* of our twelve-hour shift! I just hoped it wasn't going to be one of those days where you start as you mean to go on.

I never did follow up on Daniel's outcome, but I do know that he recovered and was discharged, because while sat in the mess room just a few weeks after Jess and I had attended to him, an emergency call was passed to a fellow paramedic and his crewmate. They were dispatched to a twenty-four year old known epileptic who was convulsing. The address given was Daniel's.

'Good luck, I hope you've had your Weetabix,' I said to the crew while laughing, anticipating the hell that, unbeknown to them, they would soon likely endure.

Chapter 6
Calved Up

Throughout most of my NHS career, I've been in and out of prison... not through any fault of my own, I hasten to add! I mean as a paramedic, attending to inmates confined to Her Majesty's Hotel.

Inmates tend to learn 'the system' pretty quickly. If they want some time out from behind the prison walls, they know that their best bet is to do something that requires a visit to the hospital, which in most cases involves an NHS ambulance being dispatched to assess, treat and, if necessary, convey them. A visit to the hospital – or what is considered by inmates a 'jolly' (I can think of better jollies myself) – is usually achieved by complaining of chest pain, abdominal pain, or by self-harm. The latter is obviously caused by mental health issues, not carried out just to guarantee a jolly, and might involve an overdose of prescription drugs, while some inmates choose to lacerate a part, or several parts, of their anatomy in order to win themselves a jolly.

Now you might be asking yourself the question, how do they get hold of prescription medication and sharp instruments? As for prescription medication, I haven't got a clue – well, I have an idea but cannot answer the question with any qualified knowledge. The answer to the second, however, sharp instruments, is they remove the blade from a shaving razor, which I assume they're allowed to have in their possession or somehow acquire, and then use a lighter to melt the blade into the head of a toothbrush. What is produced is a potentially lethal weapon to use on other inmates, or alternatively to self-harm.

Another route to a jolly is by consuming excess prison hooch, which is a potent alcoholic liquid made from apples, oranges, fruit cocktail, ketchup, sugar, milk and other ingredients, including crumbled bread. How do they get hold of the fruit to manufacture prison hooch? It's simple. They take a piece of fruit back to their cell after each 'chow time' and place it on the window sill to attract sunlight then, using illegally acquired contra-band equipment, produce prison hooch. They then drink it discreetly in their cell, becoming very drunk, very fast. Hardly 'self-harm' you may say, but at the same time they neck some prescription drugs, such as pain killers and/or anti-depressants. What the wardens are subsequently confronted by is an intoxicated, aggressive inmate hell bent on a good fight.

Whatever the method, it results in a 'jolly' outside of the confines of the prison compound, at the local A&E. There, they enjoy some alternative scenery, gawp at pretty nurses, absorb some vitamin D from the sunlight, and revel in a bit of time away from staring at the same four walls for what must feel like eternity. It's incredible what goes on inside Her Majesty's Hotels. I've even known one cell mate to insert a butternut squash into the rectum of another cell mate! That must have required some considerable force. Whether that eye-watering act was done for a jolly, sexual pleasure, self-harm or punishment, I don't know, but the very thought of it has scarred me for life, and now I'll never get to know what butternut squash tastes like!

That inmate got a jolly, whether he wanted one or not, and an x-ray for his bravery. On analysing the x-ray, the observing doctor commented that the image looked like a baby's head inside the man. He'd obviously seen some very unfortunate babies if their heads looked like a butternut squash.

That is about the limit of what I understand about the prison system. Fortunately, the prison wardens and officers know exactly what cunning tricks are attempted throughout a typical day and night amongst the jailbirds.

I remember the first time I was called to Her Majesty's Hotel as a paramedic. Although apprehensive, I was actually quite excited, which was my morbid curiosity trait emerging. Most of us have it, I'm sure. I was expecting it to be as seen in an American prison movie; you know, the State Penitentiary housing psychopaths and heavily built serial killers with that many tattoos they could be easily mistaken for a walking pop-up picture book. I always imagined a prison would have several levels, with all the walls painted brilliant white. I also imagined rows of cells with inmates gripping the bars with both hands, snarling. Fortunately though, it wasn't like that. In fact, it was almost the opposite. It was more like a scene from one of my favourite UK sitcoms, *Porridge*. The cells had steel doors, not bars, which clanked loudly when closed. The floors were buffed, very shiny, and slippery too, as I learnt at my colleague's expense! The walls were quite nicely painted, but not so brilliant white, more a dirty white. There were, however, several storeys as I'd imagined.

The inmates weren't the heavily built, tattooed psychopaths I'd envisaged either; the majority of them tended to be slim, some even quite nerdy looking, believe it or not. And then there were the old haggard type that looked like they couldn't and wouldn't harm a fly, let alone rape, burgle or kill. Today, having been 'inside' numerous times, I have a completely different perception of the nerdy, slim and old haggard types. Whenever I'm dispatched to a prison, I watch my back, and my crewmate's back too, because whether you're there to help them or not, inmates, who mostly hate authority, have been known to be uncooperative and incompliant, or to become hostile and aggressive towards ambulance personnel, regardless of wardens being close by.

Treble-nine calls to a prison are not always serious, life-threatening or an inmate's attempt at getting some 'time out'. Occasionally, the inmate doesn't want to go to hospital, even when advised to by a paramedic, while others most certainly intend to get out of prison... but in a body bag, as the following incident I attended to clearly demonstrated.

I was two-thirds of my way through a nightshift, working with an inexperienced ambulance technician called Meg. She was lovely and great to work with, but she tended to be what we in the ambulance service refer to as a 'Dr Death', pertaining to the likelihood that when you worked with her, you would be dispatched to 'proper jobs' throughout most of the shift. Proper jobs are those genuine emergencies that require a lot of paramedic intervention, and/or where the patient has time-critical features and is highly likely to deteriorate to cardiac arrest.

Meg and I were sat relaxing in the station mess room, when my hand portable radio sounded.

'Go ahead, over,' I said.

'Roger, RED call to HMP Stonecroft. Twenty-nine year old male, unresponsive; he's slashed his calves and bleeding profusely, over,' the dispatcher said.

'Calves? I would've thought he'd have done his wrists,' I said, looking at Meg, before pressing the push-to-talk button. 'Roger, understood,' I replied. So we exited the station and adopted our positions in the ambulance cab – her driving and me in the attendant's seat. Meg activated the blue lights and put her foot down.

My adrenal glands remained fast asleep for the entire journey to the prison, because some inmates are very good at pretending to be unresponsive for prison wardens who've never been taught how to recognise a fraud (no pun intended) or how to *really* check whether someone is unresponsive. And a non-medical person's definition of profuse bleeding is often different to the paramedics' definition.

When we arrived at the perimeter of the prison grounds, that's when the 'fun' began. You see, it's very easy to get into prison when you're a criminal; you just need to be found guilty of a crime. However, as an ambulance crew it's a little more difficult. Now, you may be asking yourself why it can be so difficult when a man is potentially bleeding to death. Well, let's take the following incident at HMP Stonecroft on this particular night as what I assume was standard procedure nationwide.

Firstly, Meg and I had to wait for the huge gates to open; we could have had a couple of games of tic-tac-toe together in the time that took. When the gates were open, Meg drove forward into an artificially lit security bay, applied the handbrake, put the gears in neutral and switched off the engine. Then we waited for the gates to close behind us; cue what could have been another couple of games of tic-tac-toe. Let's not forget that while this was happening, the patient was *potentially* bleeding to death. With the gates behind us now closed, a prison warden opened up the back of the ambulance, making sure it was an ambulance and not a converted get-away van, or perhaps to check that we didn't have a criminal stowed in the saloon who wanted to break back into prison.

He then came to the driver's side window, that Meg had wound down, and asked us to hand our mobile phones over. Why? Because you're not allowed to take them beyond the security bay, just in case you're a crooked ambulance man or woman intending to pass your mobile phone to an inmate so he can make calls from his cell, perhaps to contact his 'dealer', his better half or, if you've ever seen the look of prison food, maybe just to ring for a Domino's. Knowing this, I had hidden our mobile phones in the cab while en route to the call, because I tend not to trust anyone that I've only just met; doing so leaves you vulnerable to a scam, theft or much worse. So, upon the warden's request for our mobile phones, I informed him that Meg and I were two of the very few people left on this planet who do not carry a mobile phone while at work. Like all other wardens, he believed me… which is worrying.

We now had to wait for the gates in front of us to open, which would lead us to the inside of the prison grounds. After what could have been yet another couple of games, the front gates opened and a prison warden, wearing a high visibility jacket, escorted us to... the next set of gates, where another warden was waiting to open them up for us. Meg then drove through and we ambled slowly behind the escort, while the warden closed the gates behind us. That routine was repeated through another two or three sets of gates until we reached the block where the alleged profusely bleeding inmate was located.

Meg and I vacated the cab and I opened the side door and grabbed the paramedic bag, oxygen and ECG monitor. We were then escorted inside the building and along the ground floor corridor towards the inmate's cell. We could hear dozens of other inmates shouting obscenities and banging on their cell doors; the noise was horrendous. As we got closer to the open cell door, I could see a bucket load of claret had run out of the cell and into the corridor. It was one of those moments where I said, in a ventriloquist like manner, 'Ohhh shhhit! Here we go.'

Arriving at the entrance to the cell, I looked inside to find a prison warden knelt down next to the patient, who was dressed in only a t-shirt and boxer shorts. Upon him finding the haemorrhaging inmate, whose name was Luke, he had dragged him from his bed onto the floor, placed him on his side and extended his head back to afford him a patent airway. The warden had then attempted to apply direct pressure to the wounds by wrapping a bandage around each of his lacerated calves, but blood was clearly soaking through both at a rapid rate. The adrenaline immediately kicked in at the sight of what we were going to be dealing with, and the blatant seriousness of the inmate's condition. For a few seconds, Meg and I just stood there, staring at the copious amount of blood that had drained from the lacerations of his calves. There was blood all over the bed sheets, on the lower part of the wall, and on the cold concrete floor of the rather small cell.

My first thought was, 'Damn, I'm going to get blood all over my nice shiny boots.' My second thought was that the treble-nine caller's definition of profuse bleeding was the same as mine and, from what we could see, he was obviously a time-critical trauma patient. It quickly dawned on me that we'd need to get out of the block and back through all those gates and to hospital as fast as possible!

I took a deep breath to control the adrenal flow and began

thinking of my plan of action for the very pale looking patient lying in front of me. I stepped inside the cell, treading carefully around the patient who, judging by the amount of blood he'd lost and by how grey and sweaty he appeared, was evidently in hypovolaemic shock caused by a low volume of blood. His vital organs were not being adequately perfused due to an insufficient amount of oxygenated blood circulating the body. Placing the equipment down onto the cold, hard floor, I knelt down next to the warden, having no choice but to put my boots and knees into the blood on the floor. Due to the inmate's dire presentation, I immediately measured his respiratory rate and then palpated for a radial pulse in his wrist. He was breathing adequately, but there was no pulse.

The absence of a radial pulse usually signifies a systolic blood pressure below eighty millimetres of mercury, or 80mmHg, although textbook figures vary. Because Luke didn't have a palpable radial pulse, I checked for a central pulse; the carotid pulse in his neck. He had one, and it was pulsating at over 100 BPM. I wasn't overly concerned about the exact rate at this point because he was evidently in the early stages of hypovolaemic shock, so I expected his heart rate to be fast; I just wanted to ensure he had a palpable pulse. Luke's palpable carotid pulse indicated to me that his systolic blood pressure was not likely to be lower than 60mmHg, but it may not have been much higher than that either, and a blood pressure that is only just above 60mmHg would be life-threateningly low! I also immediately noted how clammy and cold to the touch he was, so cold in fact that a measurement of his sats was futile as it would have more than likely given me an inaccurate reading, so I refrained from even trying to obtain an SP02 measurement.

With initial observations undertaken within a matter of seconds, I turned to the warden and asked,

'Has he taken medication too, or just slashed his calves?' I asked inquisitively and with relevance.

'No, he's just slashed his calves, nothing else... I don't think so, anyway. I don't know, actually,' he replied indecisively.

'What time did he slash 'em, do you know? And what length and depth are the cuts?' I asked.

'We're not entirely sure, but he was fine an hour ago. The cuts are about three or four inches long and wide and deep; you can see all the muscle, tissue an' fat an' stuff. He's done a proper job with a razor blade.' I directed my gaze at Meg, still stood at the entrance to the cell.

'Right, Meg, take a warden with you and go and get the stretcher in here as fast as you can, we need to move fast,' I said with a sense of urgency in my voice. Glancing back at the warden, I said, 'Can you get another bandage on each of his calves as quick as possible, 'cause it's pissing out of him!'

Following my requests, one warden offered to assist Meg while the other began applying further dressings to Luke's calves. I began ascertaining Luke's conscious level. In the medical profession, the method used to assess a patient's consciousness level is called the 'AVPU' scale:

'A' is 'Alert'.

'V' is 'responds to Verbal stimuli'.

'P' is 'responds to Painful stimuli'.

'U' is 'Unresponsive to any stimuli'.

So, knelt down next to Luke, I put my mouth to his ear and shouted,

'Luke, can you hear me!?' No sound emerged from his mouth. 'Luke, can you hear me!?' Once again nothing emerged; Luke wasn't alert or responding to verbal stimuli. So instead, using the side of my pen torch and both my hands, I pressed hard on the nail bed of his right hand with the torch. That is usually very painful for the recipient and exactly why health care professionals use the technique as part of the AVPU, to assess for a patient's response to painful stimuli. Try it yourself if you dare. The pain usually causes you to pull away fast and shout OUCH! Luke didn't pull away, he felt nothing. It's rare but on some people that technique doesn't work, whether fully conscious or not. I had to assume he was unconscious and not one of those rare people, so I made a mental note of Luke's initial conscious level as a 'U'. Since he was unresponsive to any stimuli, I took out a nasopharyngeal airway adjunct from the paramedic bag, applied KY jelly to it and inserted it, with a slight twisting motion, into his right nostril. I then applied an oxygen mask to his face and administered high flow oxygen to him; he needed it because he'd lost a lot of the oxygen carrying blood that would normally keep his vital organs happy.

With Luke's AVPU, airway, breathing and circulation checked, I shone my pen torch into his eyes to gauge the size of his pupils. That can signify whether particular drugs have been ingested, and also to assess for the pupils' reaction to light, as that too can be a significant finding. His pupils were quite small and reacted sluggishly. 'Drugs may be the cause,' I thought. I then made a rapid mental calculation of his GCS. It was three, the lowest score possible, which confirmed he was unconscious.

To keep it really simple, a GCS is a number from three to fifteen based on a patient's consciousness level, which can fluctuate, both up and down, throughout an assessment and treatment; anything lower than fifteen is classed as a reduced level of consciousness.

Throughout the incident, the human physiology elements I'd noted while assessing Luke went back through my mind and confused me a little. Luke's signs and symptoms of excessive haemorrhaging were almost textbook-like, but his respiratory rate led me to believe that drugs of some sort had been ingested as part of his suicide plan. Rather than having an increased respiratory rate, as I'd have expected, he had a quite normal rate. Excessive haemorrhaging often causes air hunger, and the more blood lost, the greater the respiratory rate becomes. And, due to him bleeding profusely, I also expected his pupils to appear dilated, as opposed to their quite small size. Bleeding to that extent usually causes adrenaline to be secreted by the body and therefore the pupils to dilate.

This highlights the most difficult part of a paramedic's job: Maintaining the physiological knowledge and correlating that to the patient's presenting signs and symptoms, history of events and vital signs undertaken while in your care. It is even more difficult when patients don't possess the expected physiological signs and symptoms that are not only taught during training, but also from what you have read in physiology books. Fortunately, where appropriate, patients we admit into A&E have blood samples taken from them. Those tests tend to answer a lot of the diagnostic questions that paramedics cannot answer in the pre-hospital environment.

While trying not to let the noise of the shouting and banging of cell doors by other inmates distract me from my efforts to stabilise Luke, I applied the defibrillator pads to his chest and torso to enable me to monitor his heart rate using 'defib' pads alone. The ECG monitor displayed a rapid heart rate of 141 BPM. That figure, combined with an impalpable radial pulse, spoke volumes to the seriousness of Luke's condition.

My next step was to obtain IV access before he completely shut down. I applied a tourniquet to his right arm, pulling it taut to engorge the blood in his veins, and then began rummaging through the paramedic bag for a cannula. I chose a large bore cannula, primarily used on patients with life-threatening trauma injuries: It was safe to say that Luke possessed such injuries. Holding his wrist with my right hand, I used my left hand to pat the area at the fold of his right arm, where a good vein can usually be found on most patients. A hint of blue tinge appeared at the site, not a lot but enough for me to have a crack at cannulating. So, with a prepared cannula in hand, I pierced the skin with the needle. He felt nothing. I'd been hoping he would try to pull away because that would have meant his GCS had increased slightly. I waited for the flashback of blood to appear in the chamber and advanced the needle further when it did, then withdrew slightly and awaited a secondary flashback to appear along the tube's length. The secondary flashback appeared, so I unclipped the tourniquet, applied pressure and then withdrew the needle completely. Having safely disposed of the needle, I screwed the Luer-Lock to the end of the cannula and quickly secured it in place with an adhesive dressing and a net-like bandage, before flushing it with a pre-filled, ten-millilitre syringe of sodium chloride to confirm patent IV access.

'Right, I need a bag of fluid,' I said in a fast tone, thinking out loud. 'Can you wrap another bandage around each of his calves, blood is coming through again,' I said, directing my gaze at the redundant warden.

'Yeah, no problem, mate,' he replied.

While the warden did as I'd requested, and while I was waiting for Meg to return with the stretcher so that we could attempt a quick egress, I measured Luke's blood glucose level and also prepared a bag of sodium chloride to infuse through Luke's veins. This would help to restore some of the circulating fluid volume he'd lost through haemorrhaging from his self-inflicted wounds. However, when administering fluid to Luke, I had to take in to account the fact that the body has a natural defence mechanism when it senses haemorrhaging, which is to clot, exactly what I wanted his lacerations to do. But administering fluid can encourage clots to dilute and break down, therefore causing haemorrhaging to either recommence where having ceased, or it can reduce the body's own natural clotting from functioning. I made the decision to administer fluid regardless of the potential consequences; as far as I was concerned, Luke needed fluid and fast! So I attached the giving set to the cannula in Luke's arm and opened up the 'pinch', asking another warden, stood outside the cell, to come in and assist by holding the bag up. That allowed fluid to run freely and rapidly through Luke's veins, hopefully increasing his blood pressure to a level where a radial pulse could be palpated, and to a level that would buy Luke some valuable time.

By now, the warden had applied further bandages to Luke's calves, but those fresh bandages soon began to show small amounts of blood soaking through them once again. I wasn't only concerned that he'd lacerated an artery and/or vein in each calf, but also that he may have deliberately ingested blood thinning medication – such as aspirin – to aid his attempt at suicide, as the blood on the floor wasn't clotting as much as it usually does after a short period. Given the time it had taken us to get into the prison grounds and then to Luke's cell, I would have expected to see more clotted blood.

After several minutes, Meg appeared with the stretcher and positioned it outside the cell. She'd also brought the scoop stretcher to enable us to lift Luke up off the floor while keeping him horizontal, as this would minimise his blood pressure from plummeting in response to movement. That's what we chose to do and so, keeping Luke on his side, Meg positioned the scoop onto the ground, separated it and placed one half underneath him. I then rolled him the opposite way so Meg could place the other half underneath him before clipping the two ends together, forming a stretcher. Then, between Meg, the warden and I, we carefully but quickly lifted the scoop off the floor, carried it out of the cell and positioned the scoop onto the stretcher. With a warden still holding the bag of fluid up, and another warden carrying our equipment, without delay we wheeled the stretcher through the prison block. Inmates continued to shout and bang on the cell doors as we began vacating the premises.

When we reached the exit, we wheeled the stretcher up the ramp before securing it in place with the holding mechanism. Although the stretcher has a 'feature' whereby you can raise the bottom end to elevate a patient's legs, I couldn't do that on this occasion because Luke was on the scoop stretcher. For that reason, I chose to encourage an increase in Luke's blood pressure by piling several folded blankets and placing them under the foot end of the scoop, thus reducing Luke's physiological circulatory system from having to work as hard against gravity.

'Right, Meg, put a resus call in. Tell them to have 'O' negative blood on standby. We've got a twenty-nine year old male, GCS three, deep lacerations to both calves, unstable, in hypovolaemic shock. IV access secured and a fluid challenge in situ. ETA fifteen to twenty minutes,' I said with clear instruction. The reason I gave an ETA of fifteen to twenty minutes was because the time consuming security procedure doesn't change when leaving the prison, nor do the gates open quicker when you have an inmate on-board the ambulance with life-threatening injuries.

Luke was on the ambulance, accompanied by two prison wardens, and Meg had put a resus call in. We were ready to get moving, so I gave Meg the all clear to begin ambling along the route through the prison grounds. While she began to head off, I continued to monitor Luke's vital signs. His heart rate was now 136 BPM. I don't think my heart rate was far off that figure either, funnily enough, but in my case it was Luke's time-critical presentation causing adrenaline to race through my veins, and because he had the potential to deteriorate in to traumatic cardiac arrest at any time.

As we moved slowly through the prison grounds, I applied further bandages to Luke's calves and then prepared the automatic blood pressure measuring cuff. I wrapped the cuff around Luke's left arm and pressed the start button. The cuff inflated as normal and then began to deflate, which was also normal. However, it fully deflated and wouldn't display a blood pressure reading. That either meant that Luke's blood pressure was too low for the monitor to be able to make an accurate measurement, or the movement of the ambulance was causing the machine to fail. I had to assume it was because his blood pressure was too low. Under the circumstances, an exact blood pressure measurement wasn't an absolute necessity and so I would merely have to judge his status by palpable and impalpable pulse points.

While we continued to trundle through the prison grounds, I measured Luke's blood glucose level for a second time and then quickly attached another bag of fluid to the giving set, as the first bag had by now fully infused and he still had no palpable radial pulse. I was hoping the second bag, running through the cannula at full speed, would afford him at least a systolic blood pressure of 80mmHg and therefore a radial pulse to become palpable.

We had been slowly driving through the prison grounds for several minutes when we finally reached the open doors of the security bay. Once again, a warden opened up the back doors of the ambulance to check everything was legitimate, before slamming the doors shut again. Once the security doors behind us had closed, the front doors began to open. As soon as there was a large enough gap for the ambulance to fit through, Meg drove out, activated the blue lights and put her foot down in the direction of the A&E department. En route to the hospital, I continuously monitored Luke's GCS and other vital signs.

When we arrived at the A&E department, Meg parked up, swiftly vacated her seat, opened up the back doors and lowered the ramp. We quickly wheeled Luke from the ambulance, down the ramp and into the resus cubicle, where a trauma team consisting of A&E consultants, nurses and an anaesthetist were waiting for us. The team assisted Meg and I to lift Luke onto the resus bed. The consultant was waiting for my handover, which went something like this:

'Right, this is Luke, twenty-nine years old. He's slashed both of his calves with a razor blade; evidence of profuse bleeding witnessed. Warden states the lacerations are three or four inches in length, and are wide and deep.

'On arrival, Luke was in the recovery position, airway clear, but nasopharyngeal airway inserted and tolerated. Respiratory rate adequate, O2 administered. Luke appeared grey and sweaty and was cold and clammy to the touch. His calf wounds were bandaged by the warden but soaking through fast, so further bandages applied on scene and en route. There was an excessive amount of blood on the floor of the cell; difficult to gauge exact volume.

'GCS three; no change throughout. Unknown cause of why he has a GCS of three, although it's not known whether any medications have been ingested in addition to his self-inflicted injuries. His pupils are quite small and react sluggishly to light.

'Radial pulse absent, but central pulse present throughout. I was unable to measure a BP at all.

'His ECG rate is one hundred and thirty-six BPM. Blood glucose OK. Large bore IV access gained and approximately one litre of fluid administered. Are there any questions?'

'No, thank you,' the doctor replied. The team then continued to assess and treat Luke with haste, as he was a very poorly man. He also had another cannula placed in his left arm, from where blood samples were taken for clinical toxicology purposes. The wounds on his calves also received immediate attention, as blood continued to soak through the several layers of bandages that had been applied. With Luke in the expert hands of the resus team, Meg and I went outside to tidy up a little and to complete the appropriate paperwork. We then cleared from the hospital and returned to station to change our blood-stained uniform, disinfect our boots and check out a spare vehicle, as ours needed a deep clean.

A short time later, we received a further call to take an elderly patient home from the A&E department; she had fallen earlier that night but had not sustained any serious injuries. So while I was in the A&E department, I asked the doctor treating Luke what the likely outcome would be for him. He informed me that Luke was stable after receiving emergency blood, and them having located the exact site of the bleed in his calves and temporarily clamped them until he went for surgery. As a result, his blood pressure had increased and was measurable, and consequently his heart rate had decreased, too.

Upon asking the doctor what the cause of Luke's unconsciousness had been, he informed me that, although not confirmed, he highly suspected an overdose of opiate-based prescription drugs – a short time after we had cleared from A&E, a mixture of empty drugs packets had been found hidden in Luke's cell and this had been reported to the doctors caring for him. I never did find out what drugs were found exactly, but now that opiate-based drugs were suspected, Luke's bizarre presentation following his traumatic attempt at suicide began to make sense to me after all.

Chapter 7
When Your Number's Up

Throughout the earlier part of my frontline career, having made the transition from the PTS – the non-emergency aspect of the ambulance service – to the frontline emergency ambulance service as an ambulance technician, I'd be on tenterhooks waiting for the next emergency, wondering who, what, where I'd be dispatched to next. When the telephone rang or the radio sounded, I'd eagerly wait for the dispatcher to inform my crewmate and I what the nature of the emergency call was. My more experienced colleagues wouldn't be worried about what they were going to be dispatched to next, and at first I couldn't understand how they remained so relaxed during their shift.

By the time several months had passed by, I did understand and so very quickly adopted the same laid back approach to dispatchers' calls as my fellow paramedics, and have done to the present day. However, even if you don't necessarily think about what's coming next, there are those emergencies that every paramedic fears being dispatched to – seriously sick children. It is an experience I've had to endure on several occasions. This following incident was one of those occasions.

It was noon and I was sat on standby in an RRV, reading. Five minutes later, the car radio sounded.

'Go ahead, over.'

'Roger, RED call to 'Magnolia', Scotch Lane, twelve year old female, collapsed, unresponsive. Back-up crew being mobilised too, over,' the dispatcher said.

When the message was passed, my heart sank: Not because the

dispatcher had said twelve year old collapsed and unresponsive, but because she'd said 'Magnolia'. No door number, just Magnolia. I wasn't overly concerned about the nature of the call because I'd experienced numerous calls of the like, the vast majority of them having turned out to be a silly teenager pretending to be unresponsive to gain their parents' attention. I'm serious, it happens! So why did my heart sink when the dispatcher said 'Magnolia'? Well I'll explain, but firstly allow me to give you a little history lesson about house names.

Naming one's house is an old British tradition which began with affluent people naming their huge, luxurious dwellings. The tradition gradually spread and everyday people began naming their homes too. The house name would traditionally be based on who was associated with its location, or where it was. Nowadays, people name their homes from all sorts of influences, such as a feature visible on their land, like an orchard, subsequently naming their house 'The Orchards'.

Properties throughout Great Britain were allowed to have only a house name up until the mid-eighteenth century, after which time an act of Parliament ordered that all new properties, including those assigned an officially registered house name, must have a house number in addition to a street name, for ease of identifying one's address. From my experience as both a postman and a paramedic, that law is clearly not adhered to by all, because I've been to numerous houses that I'm pretty certain were built post-eighteenth century but that were identified by name only.

Now if the following explanatory, frustrated rant offends anyone then I assure you I don't intend it to, and you have my unreserved apology right now; I simply have your best interests at heart. So here we go. In my opinion, one of the most frustrating things about being a paramedic is being dispatched to an address that has a house name and no number, or in some cases, a name and a number but the treble-nine caller has provided the call-taker with the name of the house only, and then expects the swift arrival of an ambulance crew.

Finding an address with a house name in the daylight is bad enough, but in the dark, with or without street lighting, it is an absolute nightmare, let me tell you! If you're in the emergency services, particularly the ambulance or the police, you'll know exactly where I'm coming from here, but for others I imagine you may be asking, 'What's the big issue? People have house plaques on display, don't they?' Well yes, some do, and then again some don't, but whether they do or don't often makes very little difference. Why? Well, by way of example, I once asked a treble-nine caller why he didn't have a clearly identifiable house name plaque visible from the roadside. This came after I'd spent twenty minutes trying to locate his address long after I'd arrived onto the lengthy, winding road his house was located on. He answered,

'What do I need a plaque for? I know the name of my house, and I know where I live.' As the patient I'd been called to assess wasn't acutely sick and didn't present with any time-critical features, I responded to the gentleman with,

'Would you drive along in your car and, upon approaching a roundabout, fail to indicate to the person behind you what your intended exit was, because *you* know where you're going?'

'Well no, of course not, that'd be stupid, wouldn't it!' was his ignorant reply. I rest my case, I thought.

On another occasion, one Saturday or Sunday morning, I again struggled to locate an address with a house name and no number. Fortunately, it wasn't a blue light response; I'd simply been dispatched by the out-of-hours service to assess a patient with a minor condition. So I pulled over and stopped close to a gentleman who was mowing his lawn.

'Excuse me, where's 'Pier View'?' I asked.

'I don't know, mate,' he replied.

'Well, if *you* don't know, and you live on the same lane, why should I be expected to know? Why can't people just have a number on their house instead of naming it like it's their pet?' I asked him in a frustrated tone.

'What difference would it make?' he asked, frowning at me. Do I really need to explain, I thought. Yes, I obviously did, so I proceeded to explain to him.

'Well, if I'm looking for an even number, let's say number sixteen, and I can see a house with a number ten on it, then in most cases I simply have to look if the house numbers are ascending or descending to the left or the right, and then count three more houses. The majority of the time, I am highly likely to find number sixteen, aren't I?'

'It doesn't work like that round here, mate. I don't think anybody has a door number in this lane,' he replied.

'Well, it'll cost them dearly one day,' I said.

Now you might be thinking, 'the clue is in the title, Andy' and you'd be right, to a degree. Sometimes you can find an address by a little observational work; for example, 'The Beeches', so you look for a house that might have beech trees in the garden.

Then again, several houses on an estate, or along a lane, might have beech trees but a different house name, with or without a plaque, so that doesn't always help. Similarly, in the case of the house I was looking for, 'Pier View', most if not all of the houses on that particular lane would have had a view of the pier from some part of the house, albeit scarce in some cases.

With house names, you have to start at the end of the lane or road and stop at each one to check the name of it – if it has a visible plaque, that is – before moving on to the next one, checking the name of that one too, and on and on it goes. That can be very time consuming and can make the difference between life and death when responding to a potentially life-threatening incident. With numbers, you arrive on the street, lane, road, avenue etcetera, and look to your left and right to confirm which side has even numbers and which side has odd numbers. Then, with the exception of some maze-like estates, you simply follow the house numbers and very easily locate the address you're looking for. The time saved by having door numbers, compared to house names, is significant, believe me!

I remember one particular incident where my colleague and I were dispatched to a male in cardiac arrest at an address with a house name. Upon arriving on the correct lane, we couldn't locate the house. We crawled along in the ambulance, navigating the lane's entire length a couple of times but to no avail, so we stopped and asked ambulance control if they could get a relative to look out for us and provide an SOS wave. After carrying out our request, the dispatcher passed a message informing us that somebody would be outside, waving. Excellent! The call was to a cardiac arrest, after all, so we were keen to get to the patient as soon as possible. We drove along the lane again, continuing to look for the correct name plaque and also scanning the area for somebody waving, but still there was no sight of the plaque or anyone waving. We reached the opposite end of the lane once again, stopped and contacted ambulance control, informing them that nobody and no address could be located. Consequently, Control rang the treble-nine caller's telephone number, but got no answer.

We were getting rather frustrated because where we had been sat on standby, when the emergency call was passed to us, was just five minutes' drive from the lane. We went up and down the lane several more times but still had no joy. Ten minutes later, while ambling along the lane for the umpteenth time, we spotted a lady waving at us from the furthest point of a driveway that must have been forty or fifty yards long; it was huge. We couldn't believe where she was stood. To make matters worse, when we pulled up to the wrought iron gates to enter the premises, we were then delayed by the fact that they were electric gates that opened at a snail's pace... actually, a similar speed to the gates at HMP Stonecroft!

After finally accessing the property, my crewmate and I rushed into the house to find a lady performing CPR on her own husband. We worked on him for twenty minutes or so to give him the benefit of the doubt, but he was confirmed dead at the scene. What medically caused his death I don't know, possibly a heart attack, but what stood him very little chance from the moment he collapsed in cardiac arrest was not having a clearly identifiable name plaque on the wrought iron gates of his house, that I am certain!

Ambulance personnel have even heard the following many times in these circumstances after eventually arriving at the address of a treble-nine caller. On politely informing them that the delay had been caused by them being unable to find the location because they couldn't clearly see, or even find, the house name plaque, the response they received was:

'Well, we've had paramedics here before.'

Oh well, if you've had paramedics here before, and I'm a paramedic too, then I should know where it is, shouldn't I, wearing the same uniform and all that. That makes perfect sense, doesn't it? Silly me!

Here's another. Same scenario, you know, we struggled to find the address but we're now with the patient:

'The postman finds us alright!'

I used to be a postman and so I know that postmen generally get allocated a permanent delivery route, and so I would expect the postman to know where, for example, 'Rose Cottage' is, once he has found it for the first time. Unbelievable!

This final example is my most favourite of all:

'We had a fire here two years ago, it completely gutted the kitchen. The flames and smoke were sky high, they were! The Fire Service found us easy enough, though.'

'Really, I wonder how?!' I thought. Good grief, how some people think never ceases to amaze me. I'm pretty certain that there are thousands upon thousands of homeowners who adopt the same attitude as those I've experienced and described above. Then there are probably thousands upon thousands who just haven't thought about it, because they've never had to call an ambulance or any of the other emergency services in their life to date, and so haven't yet experienced the consequences of their house being identified by name only. Anyway, now I've had my rant, let's move on.

I began mobilising in the direction of Scotch Lane to the twelve year old collapsed and unresponsive. During the high speed drive, I began pondering about the house name, Magnolia. 'I wonder if the outside of the house will be painted magnolia, or should I look for magnolia trees in the garden? I don't know, I'll have to wait and see when I get to Scotch Lane,' I thought. Then the cab radio sounded,

'Go ahead, over,' I said, using the hands-free PTT button that's situated centimetres from the steering wheel.

'Roger, update for you. You are responding to a twelve year old cardiac arrest. Back-up remaining en route, over,' the dispatcher said.

'Shit!' I thought, but replied with, 'Roger, understood, over.' Adrenaline kicked in immediately. My stomach churned and my heart rate doubled in seconds. Due to the potential nature of the call, I added a little more weight to the accelerator pedal to arrive on scene a little quicker, doing my utmost best to concentrate on my emergency driving standard and not think too much, if at all, about what I might be dealing with in a couple of minutes time. I say 'might be dealing with' because it may have still turned out to be what is known in the ambulance service as *'Not as given'*.

When I arrived on Scotch Lane, I turned the sirens off and slowed the vehicle right down to an amble, alternately casting my eyes on the road and at any visible house name plaques on the left and right side, looking for 'Magnolia', but no joy. I gave a short burst of the siren to try to prompt somebody from the correct address to come outside. Unusually, that didn't work. I gave a second short burst of the siren to prompt attention. Still no joy! 'Maybe they're doing CPR,' I thought. So I continued to crawl along the lane, squinting to read the plaques on the walls of houses and on the gates, some of which were in such a poor state that they were useless.

I continued this for a further few minutes, periodically sounding short bursts from the siren. I was beginning to feel a little annoyed with the situation and the problems that house names bring, and the difference they can make between life and death. As if the adrenaline from getting the call in the first place wasn't bad enough, the situation was increasing the adrenal flow through my body. I gave another blast of my siren as a last ditch attempt at gaining attention before contacting Control and asking them to get someone out to me. Then a figure appeared ahead, a lady waving at me with a cordless telephone in her hand, held to her ear. Unbeknown to me at that time, she was being given CPR instructions by an ambulance control room call-taker, and had been conveying those instructions to her husband prior to coming outside to flag me down. As she appeared extremely upset, I began to think that this call was going to be a genuine paediatric cardiac arrest after all. I quickly drove up to the distraught lady, hastily exited the RRV and hurriedly grabbed my equipment from the saloon. As I promptly followed the lady through the gate and towards the front doorway, I heard sirens approaching close by. 'At least they'll find the address easy enough, now my car is outside of it,' I thought as I entered the house.

'Where's the patient?' I asked, with a little tremor in my voice.

'In the lounge, he's doing CPR on her,' the lady said, crying inconsolably. My heart beat became progressively faster as I walked through the house, with equipment to hand, ready to face every paramedic's worst nightmare. Whether the patient is twelve weeks old or twelve years old, it doesn't matter – attending to a seriously sick, injured or dead child is very upsetting. With the exception of a major incident, it's as stressful as it can possibly get!

I rushed into the lounge to find the youngster lying flat on her back. From her moribund appearance, she was evidently in cardiac arrest. As stated by the distraught lady, the young girl's dad was performing chest compressions, so I immediately knelt down on the carpeted floor at her head end.

'What's happened, does she have any medical problems at all?' I asked her distressed dad.

'No, she just stood up and collapsed,' he informed me, continuing compressions.

'OK, let me take over, you go and comfort your wife. I'll do my best, and I've got more help on the way,' I instructed empathetically. While it is sometimes helpful for a bystander who has commenced chest compressions to continue when there is only a solo paramedic on scene, I decided that in this case it was too traumatising for this young girl's dad. More importantly, his distress was causing his rate and depth of compressions, and the placement of his hands, to be ineffective and so counter-productive if she had any chance of being successfully resuscitated. He came to his feet, sobbing his heart out. I heard him uttering a name as he left the room,

'Hannah… Hannah.'

That was a very sombre moment.

Nevertheless, I had to crack on. So with my heart going like the clappers, I swiftly cut Hannah's upper garments off then rapidly applied the defibrillator pads and switched the machine on. My intention was to view her heart rhythm through the pads, and 'shock' her if appropriate. Although children in cardiac arrest rarely present with a 'shockable' rhythm, they do occur from time to time. The monitor beeped and I waited a second or two for her heart rhythm to display. Sadly, a flatline rhythm appeared on the screen. Her heart wasn't beating slowly or in an uncoordinated manner, as it does when VF is present. It had stopped beating altogether. From that moment, regardless that my imminently arriving crewmates and I would do our utmost best for Hannah, I knew that day was going to be a very sad day indeed.

I'm not a pessimistic man, my glass is generally always half-full, but I just knew that flatline rhythms seldom restore to a rhythm compatible with life. I'd attempted resuscitation on hundreds of patients presenting in the same rhythm, and I could count on *one hand* how many were initially successful, but not in the long-term. I also knew that fit and healthy children don't just collapse and die without an underlying medical problem. Whatever undiagnosed medical condition Hannah had, my only hope was that, because she was young, she might respond to treatment. So, with equipment by my side, I began compressing her chest at a rate of one hundred times per minute, momentarily pausing to grab the BVM. I quickly attached it to an oxygen cylinder, extended her neck to open her airway, and then squeezed two artificial ventilations into her mouth, before recommencing effective chest compressions.

As I was performing compressions, two of my colleagues

141

entered the lounge, so I began delegating tasks.

'Right, John, carry on with compressions and check the monitor every two minutes,' I requested.

'OK, mate,' John replied, obviously distressed by the age of the patient.

'Bill, you get a line in and give her some adrenaline as quick as you can, mate.'

'OK. Are you gonna intubate?'

'Yeah, then we need to think about gettin' out of here,' I replied. In the background, all we could hear while resuscitating Hannah was hysterical screaming and crying. It is by far one of the most difficult scenarios a paramedic can find themselves in.

A further five minutes passed and by now Bill had obtained IV access and had commenced drug therapy. John was performing continuous compressions, and I had managed to get a tube down her windpipe and had attached her to the automatic ventilator, therefore leaving my hands free. That gave me the opportunity to obtain a blood glucose measurement and set up a bag of fluid to attach to the cannula in her arm. It also gave me the opportunity to consider the reasons why she had collapsed and was in cardiac arrest.

As part of the Advanced Life Support (ALS) algorithm, resuscitation providers – in our case paramedics – have to consider what is known as the four H's and four T's in order to rule in or rule out a cause of cardiac arrest. This is also used to decide whether we can clinically intervene and increase the patient's chance of survival. Now don't worry, I'm not going to even begin to explain the four H's and four T's to you – as a layperson reading this, it would blow your mind – but what I will say is that during this particular incident, we were pretty much able to eliminate most of the H's and T's. That led us to believe that the likely cause of Hannah collapsing in cardiac arrest was due to an unknown abnormality in her heart, which may have caused a sudden abnormal rhythm, not compatible with life, to occur without warning. It had to be; there was no reason to suggest drugs or poisoning, she wasn't hypothermic, and her blood sugar levels were normal. There was no trauma involved and she had no significant past medical history whatsoever. As far as Hannah and her family were concerned, she had been as fit and healthy as any typical, carefree, pretty young girl.

Unfortunately, Hannah had remained in a flatline rhythm throughout the resuscitation thus far, with no signs of life at all. Nevertheless, we intended to convey her through to hospital, continuing with advanced life support measures throughout the entire journey to A&E, and for a while longer in the department, too. So, keen to get Hannah into the ambulance and rush her to hospital, I took over compressions while John went out to the ambulance to fetch the scoop and the stretcher. When he returned, Bill and I rolled Hannah to one side and placed half of the scoop underneath her, then rolled her the opposite way and positioned the other half before clipping the two ends together, minimising any interruption in compressions during the course of the manoeuvre. Following that, I went to explain to Hannah's distraught parents that they could either travel with us, if they so wished, or if it was understandably too traumatising to witness, then they could drive to hospital in their own car. They chose the latter, so I emphasised that we would be conveying Hannah under emergency driving conditions and therefore not to try to keep up with us. I also stressed the importance that they drove as safely as they possibly could under such difficult circumstances. With that brief discussion over, we quickly lifted the scoop with Hannah secured, hastily wheeled the stretcher out of the house, and loaded her into the saloon of the ambulance.

I'd decided to leave the RRV at the address and assist Bill throughout the journey to A&E. John had requested ambulance control to pre-alert the A&E department of the twelve year old cardiac arrest they'd be imminently receiving, and was now driving as fast and as safely as possible, taking into account that we'd be attempting to sustain effective chest compressions, which can be very difficult to perform in a moving ambulance. When we arrived at A&E, John abruptly parked the vehicle. A nurse flung the rear doors open and lowered the ramp, allowing us to rush Hannah into the resuscitation department. While lifting the scoop over to the hospital bed, unclipping each half and removing it from underneath Hannah, I gave a very brief handover while a nurse took over compressions. My handover went something like this:

'This is twelve year old Hannah. She was seen to collapse at home while at rest at approximately noon. On arrival, she was receiving CPR from her dad. Pads applied and initial rhythm was a flatline. BLS continued until back-up arrived, and then advanced measures were carried out, including intubation and drug and fluid therapy.

'No drugs or poisoning suspected. She's not hypothermic. Her blood glucose is normal, and she has no significant past medical history. She's normally fit and well.

'She's remained in a flatline rhythm throughout the entire resuscitation attempt. Are there any questions?'

'How long has she been 'down' for now?' the doctor asked.

'Approximately forty minutes, doc,' I replied.

The resus team continued with the ALS algorithm. There wasn't anything else the doctors could do that my crewmates and I hadn't already done. We remained at A&E for a little longer, periodically walking into the resus room to see if there was any change in cardiac rhythm. There wasn't. By the time the doctors had given her all benefit of the doubt, Hannah had been in cardiac arrest for nearly one hour. Sadly, they confirmed her dead.

Her parents were sat in the relatives' room, still unaware of the resus team's decision to cease attempts at trying to save Hannah's life. With Hannah having no medical history, they were obviously hoping that their daughter would respond to treatment. That hope was shattered when a consultant had the unfortunate task of going to inform them. Although I'd heard it many times before, the hysterical cries that came from the relatives' room was enough to make you want to quit and do a job that is less stressful, and one that requires a lot less responsibility.

Bill, John and I went outside and that is when I sat on the back step of the ambulance, with my head in my hands and a bucket full of adrenaline still hurtling through my veins, and thought, 'I'm not sure if I can do this anymore.' After pondering over my future career options for a little while, we vacated the grounds of the A&E department and Bill and John gave me a lift back to the RRV.

While stood by the RRV, I had a look for the house name plaque. I looked on the front of the house, the gate, even for a sign sticking out of the garden, but no, there was no sign displayed anywhere. With Hannah still on my mind, I couldn't help but despair. I drove back to the ambulance station, closely following behind Bill and John's ambulance.

Historically, when ambulance personnel have attended to the death of a child or other distressing incident, they are understandably offered some downtime back at the ambulance station, to reflect, discuss and even to cry and express their emotions, if they feel the need. The ambulance service does have counsellors in place for events like the one we'd dealt with, but while utilised by some members of staff, the majority find counsel in either the crewmate they were working with at the time of the traumatising, sad or tragic incident, or another member of ambulance staff; or sometimes amongst their own loved ones.

Several days later, following a post-mortem examination, a consultant who had been involved with the resuscitation of Hannah arranged a debrief session for all those involved, excluding her parents of course – they would be notified of the cause of Hannah's death more formally. It was confirmed that Hannah had collapsed and died from a condition known as Hypertrophic Cardiomyopathy (HCM), which is a form of heart muscle disease where the lower muscular walls of the heart – the ventricles – become abnormally thickened. Cardiomyopathy is a common congenital heart disorder that causes various heart problems, one of which is sudden death during vigorous exertion, but where death can also occur without warning during minimal exertion or even at rest, as was the case with Hannah.

But perhaps most pointedly, patients who collapse with undiagnosed HCM do so because the heart develops an arrhythmia, and in a lot of cases that arrhythmia is VF or pulseless VT, a scenario in which defibrillation is an appropriate form of medical intervention, as mentioned earlier. Though we'll never know whether Hannah's heart developed VF or pulseless VT when she initially collapsed, I couldn't help but think, what if I'd not had difficulty finding her address and had arrived at her side more promptly, and she *had* presented in VF or pulseless VT? Early defibrillation might have restored her heart to a normal rhythm compatible with life. That would have allowed us to rapidly convey Hannah to hospital so doctors could have undertaken further assessments on her, including an echocardiogram, diagnose HCM and subsequently treat her accordingly. It's obviously a lot more sophisticated than that, but what if...?

Unfortunately, a year or so later, I found myself resuscitating a fit and healthy fourteen year old girl who had collapsed in cardiac arrest while having a shower. After providing Advanced Life Support (ALS) measures for nearly an hour in total, she was confirmed dead at hospital. Sadly, following her post-mortem examination, it was confirmed that she too had died from undiagnosed Hypertrophic Cardiomyopathy (HCM).

There is a moral behind the above true account, the moral being that a poorly signed or missing house name or number could contribute to your death, or that of a loved one. If you're one of those people with either an officially registered house name, or an officially registered house name with an allocated number as well, then ask yourself the following questions:

Do you have a house name plaque?

Has the plaque become hidden behind overgrown shrubs or foliage?

If wooden, is it rotting?

Has the name been engraved only, or has the engraved title also been clearly painted?

Whatever material your plaque is made from, is the font clear and large enough to be seen from the roadside in the daylight and in the dark?

More importantly, if you had to call the emergency services today, could *you* be blamed for a significant delay in them finding your address? If you could then please, please, please act on it as soon as possible, because it might just make the difference between the life and death of yourself or a loved one!

Chapter 8
Time-Critical

OAPs... I love 'em, they're great, and they make up a fair majority of the treble-one and treble-nine incidents that ambulance personnel attend to, for obvious reasons. They're also the subject of many of the countless anecdotal stories that I can recall. For instance, I was called to attend to an elderly lady who had fallen at home. On my arrival, I found her lying flat on her back on the lounge floor of her bungalow, being cared for by three of her elderly friends. Together, they were like Blanche, Rose, Dorothy and Sophia, the old dears from the US sitcom, *The Golden Girls*. They were as funny as them too.

Fortunately, my patient hadn't lay there for long, as I'd been dispatched to her shortly after she'd fallen. I knelt down next to her and asked her not to move until I'd assessed her... well, *shouted* for her not to move, as she was as deaf as a post. I wanted to ensure she'd not potentially fractured the ball and socket joint of her hip bone – better known as the neck of femur – which is a common occurrence in the elderly following a fall. So I then began by ascertaining her name.

'Hello, my name's Andy, I'm a paramedic. What's your name, flower?' I asked. Straining her eyes while looking at *Blanche*, she shouted,

'What de'say?!'

'I said, what's your name?!'

'Eh, what de'say?!' she repeated. Moving a little closer to her, I said,

'What's your name, petal?!' With her nose scrunched and eyes squinting, she bellowed,

'What de'say, do I live on my own?!' *Rose,* despairing, yelled,

'*Sophia*, tell him your name!' Laughing, I said to *Rose*,

'Is her name *Sophia*, by any chance?'

'Yeah, have you been to her before?' she asked with interest.

'No, you fool, you've just called her by her name!' I said, chuckling. The Golden Girls giggled to themselves, with the exception of *Sophia*; bless her, she still didn't have a clue what we were talking or laughing about.

On another occasion, I attended to an elderly chap named Brian, who had fallen while stood under a bus shelter, waiting for the number five. He reminded me of *Compo* from the UK sitcom, *Last of the Summer Wine*; you know, the scruffy little sod. After a thorough check-up in the back of the ambulance to make sure he had actually fallen and not collapsed, and to ensure there were no underlying causes for the fall, I informed him that he didn't need a visit to the A&E department, which he was pleased about. Before I could let him on his way though, I had to complete the non-conveyance forms, and therefore went about ascertaining some personal details from him. Part of that conversation went something like this:

'So, your first name is Brian, is that right?' I asked to reconfirm.

'Yes, that's right,' he answered.

'OK, is that Brian with an 'I' or a 'Y'?' I asked. He thought about it for a second and then looked at me with a confused expression,

'With a 'B',' he answered. Unbelievable! I did eventually complete my documentation and assisted Brian from the ambulance and back to the bus shelter, from where I assume he got home safely.

Attending to old dears is often a giggle – though it can also be mildly frustrating – especially while trying to determine their perceived pain score. It's like trying to draw blood from a stone. The conversation is often similar to the following:

'So, Fred, about your abdominal pain, on a scale of zero to ten, how would you score your pain right now? Zero being no pain and ten being the worse pain you have *ever* been in.'

'Er… well, I've had worse.'

'OK, how would you score it now though, zero to ten?'

'Er… well, I fell and broke my wrist last year; that did hurt, I tell you. It's not as bad as that though.'

'Yeah, OK, but zero to ten, how is your abdominal pain?'

'Well, if I keep still, it's less painful than when I move.'

'Zero to ten, Fred, zero to ten?'

'I'm not sure really. It's probably more than a two.'

'Maybe a three then, Fred?'

'No, no, it's more than a three. Probably between four and six, I'd say.'

'Fred, should I put five down?'

'Yeah, yeah, it's about that, yeah.'

I'll say it again, old people, I love 'em, and I always have plenty of time for each one that I attend to. In fact, when a visit to the hospital isn't required, I frequently stick around on scene for a short time to make them a brew and have a chat about the history of their lives. The vast majority of them have some fascinating stories to tell – believe me, you'd be astonished!

This next incident involved a seventy-six year old lady who, one morning, experienced symptoms which she had never in her life experienced before.

It was a hot summer's day and I was sat on standby with my crewmate, Josh, an Emergency Care Assistant (ECA). The role, and even the title of an ECA equivalent, differs between each individual ambulance service around the UK, but regardless of the different job titles, they're very similar to Ambulance Technicians. Unfortunately, they don't receive the same level of training as a technician and therefore don't possess the same skills. ECAs (or equivalent) were a so-called 'money saving initiative', as less training, skill and responsibility means they don't have to be paid as much as a technician. For that cost-saving reason, technicians have gradually been phased out throughout the majority of the UK ambulance service, though it wouldn't surprise me if they go full circle and are one day re-introduced as part of an ambulance crew. Having said all that, the ECAs I've worked alongside have been extremely professional and are a vital asset to the frontline ambulance service.

At 9:05 a.m., the cab radio sounded.

'Receiving, over,' Josh said.

'Roger, RED call to Happy Holidays Caravan Park, to a seventy-six year old female experiencing shortness of breath. You'll be met at the entrance, over.'

'Roger, understood,' Josh replied, and with that began mobilising to the location given, using blue lights and sirens for the relatively short journey. On arriving at the entrance to the caravan site, we were met by a staff member from the park. As the park was like a maze, I stepped out of the ambulance and asked her to ride in the cab, while I got into the saloon, so she could guide Josh to the exact location of the patient's caravan. Josh followed her knowledgeable directions and, after five minutes of driving slowly around the twists and turns of the tarmacked site, we arrived at the caravan. I vacated the saloon, picked up the equipment and walked briskly towards the door already opened for our anticipated arrival.

Ascending the two metal steps, we wandered inside the caravan and there we were met by the patient's husband, and another couple who were sharing the same caravan. I walked further inside, to where the patient was situated, and was presented with a rather large lady sat in a tripod-like position on the sofa, extremely distressed. She was leant forward, supporting her upper body by placing a hand on each thigh, breathing very fast and therefore shallow. Her face was pale and extremely swollen, so much so that her eyes were being squeezed shut as if she'd done two rounds with *Mike Tyson*. Her tongue was so enlarged that it was being involuntarily forced out of her mouth, and her lips were swollen like a pouting puffer fish. Her hands, particularly her fingers, were twice their normal size, a sure sign of angio-oedema.

Normally, the immune system protects the body by detecting bacteria in the blood and produces white blood cells that destroy them. Angio-oedema is caused by the immune system incorrectly reacting to *harmless* substances in the blood.

Consequently, the body produces a chemical called histamine which causes the blood vessels in the area to expand, leading the deeper layers of the skin to puff up. The areas affected are usually the eyes, lips and hands, but it can affect any part of the body. Common causes of angio-oedema are an allergic reaction to a known source, such as nuts or shell fish. Sometimes the source is unknown and goes undetected, a condition better known as idiopathic angio-oedema.

Due to how our patient presented, Josh, recognising that she was time-critical, immediately opened the paramedic bag and attached the sats probe to her swollen index finger. Meanwhile, I crouched down beside her and introduced us both to the understandably frightened lady, taking in to account that she could barely see us, or anybody else, because her eyes were forced almost shut by the swelling. I learned from her concerned husband that my patient's name was Doris and so proceeded to inform her of what Josh and I were going to do.

'Doris, Josh is going to put a type of oxygen mask on your face in a minute, that'll help your breathing,' I said, simultaneously feeling for a pulse in her neck. It was going very fast, so fast in fact that it was impossible to count an accurate rate. There was no point in asking Doris any questions as she wouldn't have been able to clearly answer them due to the swelling of her tongue, mouth and face in general. I therefore relied on her husband, who was by now in tears out of concern for his wife.

'Is she gonna be alright?' he asked, tearfully.

'Don't worry, we'll look after her, but I need some information from you. Now, is Doris allergic to anything at all?'

'No, not that I know of,' he answered with a concerned

expression.

'OK, has she eaten anything that she's never eaten before or only had once or twice before? Or something she's not had for some considerable time?' The reason that was a significant question is because people sometimes become allergic to food stuff they've been eating for years, or haven't eaten for a long period of time.

'No, not at all,' he said, anxiously.

'Is she on any medication?'

'She's got high blood pressure, so she's on something for that. Why does it matter? Just please help her.'

It did matter, because one of the drugs I planned on administering to Doris meant that half doses should be given if on medication for high blood pressure, unless there is profound low blood pressure. With that information noted, I glanced at the sats monitor; it read eighty-nine percent. That was low. The fact that her tongue was swollen and sticking out in a child-like manner meant that her airway was narrowing, thus preventing a sufficient amount of oxygen from being inhaled and entering her lungs. If it continued to narrow and completely closed, then no air would enter at all and she would eventually collapse in cardiac arrest. Had that happened in a pre-hospital environment, there would have been absolutely nothing Josh and I could have done for her. Intubation would have been futile because there'd be no viewable, open vocal chord and, from a paramedical point of view, I'd have had no means whatsoever of adequately ventilating her.

Paramedics do possess a skill whereby they insert a cannula into the windpipe from the outside of the throat, but don't confuse that with intubation, which is a different skill altogether. The paramedic skill I'm referring to is called Needle Cricothyroidotomy. It is only an appropriate intervention if the patient is still breathing for themselves, and is only used to oxygenate a patient with an airway obstruction.

Doris remained unable to converse with me because of the severe swelling to her lips and tongue, and her breathing remained shallow. Fortunately, Josh had by now prepared a nebulised mask that has an acorn-like attachment on it, and had added a drug called Salbutamol in liquid form into the 'acorn'. When the nebuliser mask is attached to an oxygen cylinder and set between six to eight litres per minute, it produces a vapour that the patient inhales. The effect of this particular drug encourages the smooth tissue lining of the airway and lungs to relax, resulting in dilation of airway passages and a marked increase in oxygen entering the blood stream.

So with the nebuliser prepared, Josh placed the mask on to her face then went outside to fetch the carry-chair. Meanwhile, I measured her blood pressure, using the manual technique as opposed to the automatic method. I wrapped the blood pressure cuff around her left arm and inflated it. I then placed my stethoscope just over the pulse point located at the front of the elbow, near the base of the bicep muscle. After several seconds of deflating the cuff and listening for the appropriate sounds, I obtained a systolic blood pressure measurement of just 87mmHg. That was low, but combined with her rapid pulse rate it made sense to me. I strongly believed, from Doris's visual presentation, blood pressure and pulse rate, that she wasn't simply having a severe reaction to an unknown source, she was suffering from idiopathic anaphylactic shock; and by far the worst case of anaphylactic shock I had ever seen.

Like other forms of shock, anaphylactic shock can kill within minutes if not treated with the utmost urgency. As it was a time-critical, life-threatening emergency, I didn't want to hang around on scene for too long, as even with our treatment on scene she could have responded to it slowly or not at all and therefore have deteriorated rapidly. Doris was being nebulised but no significant signs of improvement were yet evident, as it needs several minutes to take effect, particularly on the quality of breathing. On the other hand, the sats percentage can and often does increase within a minute or so.

While I waited for Josh to return, I opened the drugs bag and selected an ampoule of adrenaline to inject into her thigh. By administering adrenaline to Doris, I was hopeful that it would cause her blood vessels to constrict and therefore increase her blood pressure, thus preventing her from deteriorating. If effective, it would also assist what the nebuliser was intended to do and open up her airway passage too, allowing her to breathe normally as opposed to breathing shallow.

Doris's husband and friends looked on, extremely concerned by her never-before-seen signs and symptoms. While I continued to reassure them all, including Doris, and prepared the ampoule of adrenaline, Josh returned. He'd had to leave the carry-chair just outside the entrance, because the caravan doors were very narrow. Before assisting Doris towards the carry-chair, I explained that I would need to expose a small area of her thigh to give her the adrenaline injection, and that this would hopefully begin to reduce the facial swelling and improve the quality of her breathing, along with increasing her blood pressure. Doris nodded to acknowledge that she understood and consented to the treatment. So I cleaned the area of her thigh with a little alcohol swab, pulled her skin taught and injected 250 micrograms of adrenaline into the muscle. The normal dose was 500 micrograms, but because she was on an anti-hypertensive, and because I didn't consider a systolic blood pressure of 87mmHg as profound, I chose to give her a half-dose initially, with a view to administering a further dose following a second set of observations.

Assisting her from the sofa, with the nebuliser still providing Doris with therapeutic vapour, she came to her feet. We slowly descended the steps out of the caravan, followed closely by her husband, and assisted her onto the chair, wrapped a blanket around her and secured her with straps. With haste, we then proceeded to the ambulance and encouraged Doris to position herself semi-recumbent on the stretcher, offering her worried husband a seat before continuing with further observations and treatment.

'Right mate, can you set up some IV hydrocortisone, IV chlorphenamine and a bag of fluid, while I get some obs?' I asked Josh.

'Yeah, will do, mate,' he said as he re-opened the drugs bag. That may sound like a lot of tasks to give one ECA, but that is their 'bread and butter'. Once you become a paramedic, you're less likely to prepare drugs yourself, not because it's beneath you – certainly not – but because a paramedic is usually too busy gaining IV access, intubating, interpreting ECGs or simply asking the patient numerous questions. Having said that, it depends which service you're employed by, as some services don't allow ECAs to prepare drugs for paramedics, the theory being that whoever is responsible for administering drugs should be responsible for preparing them, too. It makes sense, I suppose.

With Doris becoming more and more tired and distressed on the stretcher, I wrapped the automatic blood pressure cuff around her arm and pressed the start button. While that was inflating, I pin-pricked her finger for a drop of blood, to check her blood sugar level. I then wired her up to the ECG monitor and also prepared the cannulation equipment – if she arrested on me due to shock, I'd need patent IV access. On the other hand, if she arrested on me because her airway closed and she stopped breathing, IV access would have been as useful to me and her as a chocolate fire guard!

Glancing at the ECG monitor, I noted her heart rate of 152 BPM. That was fast and not ideal for a seventy-six year old to sustain for a prolonged period. Her second systolic blood pressure reading appeared on the monitor, it read 96mmHg. The slight improvement was a good sign, but she wasn't stable enough yet!

I'd placed the cannulation equipment on the drop-down cupboard door providing a makeshift work surface. Then, with difficulty due to Doris being a 'bonnie lass', I cannulated her right arm, securing it in place. Josh had by now prepared the IV hydrocortisone, IV chlorphenamine – *a.k.a* piriton, an anti-histamine drug – and a bag of fluid. Wasting no time, I attached the giving set to the cannula and allowed the contents to run freely, thus increasing her blood pressure. That in theory would also reduce the speed of her pulse rate, as the heart would no longer have to pump blood quite as fast as it was around her body in order to sustain an adequate systolic measurement. As the fluid challenge was in place, I informed Doris that I was going to administer hydrocortisone – a steroidal drug, the purpose of which is to reduce the substances released in the body that cause inflammation during an allergic response. In addition, I'd administer piriton and a second dose of adrenaline into her thigh muscle. Once again, Doris consented with a nod.

As her husband looked on, fortunately a little calmer as he was now seeing Doris receive treatment, Josh passed me the prepared syringe containing hydrocortisone. Manually pinching the tubing of the fluid giving set, I pushed 200 milligrams through the injection port, before releasing my pinch to allow fluid to flush the drug through. Then Josh passed me the piriton, so I once again pinched the tubing and pushed 10 milligrams of that drug through her veins too, before letting go of the pinch, allowing fluid to flow. Pinching the tube is done to prevent the drug you're administering from backing-up into the bag of fluid, therefore causing the drug to either be administered at a slower rate or, potentially, very little of it at all if the giving set is later intentionally detached from the cannula by a doctor while the patient is in hospital.

The IV drugs were in. Now I needed to give Doris a second dose of adrenaline and so injected her with a further 250 micrograms into her thigh muscle. We were ready to commence the blue light journey to A&E, with a pre-alert an absolute necessity.

During the twenty minute journey to hospital, I measured Doris's blood pressure twice more, noting an improvement and a reduced heart rate as a consequence of the treatment administered. Her quality of breathing began to improve, too. Her swollen lips had decreased in size, but still resembled those of a pouting puffer fish. Her tongue was still larger than normal but a reduction, and therefore an improvement, was noted. Doris had received the same drugs as a doctor would generally administer, but if the improvements I was witnessing reversed and the patient developed signs of a secondary reaction – a condition known as a biphasic response – then the doctor might choose to administer additional doses.

Upon arriving at the A&E department and transferring Doris onto the hospital bed, I proceeded to convey to the awaiting consultant my observational findings and a summary of the treatment provided.

'This is seventy-six year old Doris. Approximately one hour ago, she began to experience shortness of breath and her husband noticed her face beginning to swell. No known allergies recorded.

'On our arrival, Doris was GCS fifteen but unable to talk. She was pale and breathing shallow. Her sats were initially eighty-nine percent on air.

'Initial BP was eighty-seven systolic, which increased to ninety-six, and the latest measurement was one hundred and five. Her initial pulse rate was one hundred and fifty-two BPM. That has since decreased to one hundred and twenty-nine following treatment.

'Doris was given a five milligram Salbutamol NEB, and five hundred micrograms of adrenaline in two doses, plus two hundred milligrams of hydrocortisone and ten milligrams of piriton, pushed through with a fluid challenge. Any questions?'

The doctors and nurses then continued with the assessment and treatment of Doris, while her still anxious husband waited for news in the admission waiting area. Following the completion of my paperwork and restocking my drugs bag with replacement ampoules of all the drugs I'd used, Josh and I cleared from the hospital and were immediately given a further treble-nine call.

Later that day, while admitting another patient to hospital, Josh and I went to see Doris and her husband in the A&E cubicle. She was still wired up to an ECG and automatic blood pressure machine. Fortunately though, the swelling to her face, lips and tongue had reduced considerably. Her breathing was back to a normal rate, as too was her blood pressure and heart rate. She was on the road to a full recovery, but the doctors wanted to monitor and assess her for further improvement, and to ensure a repeat of the same signs and symptoms didn't occur.

After being discharged, Doris would most likely have been referred for specialist tests to try to establish a cause of her severe, life-threatening reaction. If no cause was found, she would have likely been prescribed what is known as an 'Epi-pen'. A UK Epi-pen usually contains an adult dose of 300 micrograms of adrenaline that can be self-administered in the event an anaphylactic reaction occurs, whether the patient is aware of their trigger allergy or not. Unfortunately, health care professionals, both pre-hospital and in-hospital, cannot save the life of everybody who experiences a severe allergic reaction and deteriorates to anaphylactic shock. Sadly, approximately 20 people a year die in the UK from the condition. In about half of these cases, there is no known cause.

Chapter 9
A Question of Ethics

What are ethics?

The subject of ethics is a 'minefield' to discuss, so I'm going to keep it brief, very brief. Ethics is the study of morality, and morality is a fundamental part of all our lives. We're frequently thinking and making judgements about what we should and shouldn't do, and also about what others should and shouldn't do. Even when we don't think of ourselves as morally high-minded people, we usually turn out to have strong views about the rightness or wrongness of at least some of the things that human beings do. Is it right or wrong to have an abortion? Should euthanasia be legalised around the globe? These are just a couple of the questions discussed and debated when the subject of ethics is raised.

It is well-known that the work of ambulance personnel means that they attend to patients in cardiac arrest and, therefore, frequently deal with death during their career. Fortunately, the vast majority of deaths ambulance personnel deal with are patients who are elderly. However, what age is considered 'elderly'? Seventy, seventy-five, eighty, eighty-five years old – it's subjective, isn't it?

As previously highlighted in this book, people of varying age, not just the elderly, develop medical conditions, whether known or unknown, which can cause life-threatening arrhythmias and subsequent cardiac arrest. Sometimes, cardiac arrest occurs due to a traumatic injury or injuries. When cardiac arrest occurs, whether through medical or traumatic circumstances, paramedics usually, though not always, intervene with advanced resuscitative measures. Some patients, however, are found deceased in their home by a carer and/or relative. In a lot of those incidences there is pathological evidence to suggest that the deceased has been dead for some considerable time, and so resuscitative measures would be futile and therefore are not commenced.

In other incidences, where the patient is terminally ill, an estimated period of time left to live is known by the patient and their nearest and dearest, and so death is anticipated. Therefore, the patient's dying wishes are usually planned well in advance. The patient has, in *most* of those cases, signed a valid *Advanced Decision to Refuse Treatment* (ADRT), also known as a 'Living Will', which is usually, though not always, readily available for the attending ambulance crew to view on arrival at the deceased or dying patient's side. Alternatively, or in addition to the ADRT, the patient may have signed a valid *Do Not Attempt Cardiopulmonary Resuscitation* (DNACPR) form; again this is usually, though not always, readily available to view.

Where a patient no longer possesses the mental capacity to make informed decisions for themselves – for example, if they have severe dementia – they will have usually appointed a person to act as their *Lasting Power of Attorney* (LPoA) while they had the mental capacity to do so. An LPoA can be invoked to make informed decisions on behalf of the patient.

The exception to the aforementioned is when the GP has signed the DNACPR form on the patient's behalf. This is usually known to the patient's next-of-kin or closest relatives, but not always known to the patient. You may think that is morally wrong, but it is only done because the patient no longer has the mental capacity to make informed decisions for him/herself, perhaps due to severe dementia. In that case, a GP will sign the DNACPR form if they have a good, informed reason to believe that, based on the patient's medical condition/s, CPR would either be unsuccessful or, if CPR was successful, then the result would leave the patient with subsequent severe health problems, such as brain damage, prolonged suffering or very little or no quality of life.

However, where a patient possesses either of the above mentioned signed legal documents but *does not* have them readily available to view – for instance, if they were out in public and collapsed in cardiac arrest in the street, but the documents were in their home – then paramedics are, strictly speaking, obliged to intervene with resuscitative measures against the patient's wishes. With the layperson being unaware of this obligation, I've known paramedics to have received verbal abuse in the street from a hostile member of a patient's family when intervening. You may think it is immoral for paramedics to intervene, but if the family are not able to produce a valid document, or are unable to find it anywhere in the patient's house, then where's the proof that the document actually exists or is still valid? Its review date may have expired, thus making it invalid. What's more, Living Wills and DNACPR forms can be withdrawn at any time by the patient, an attorney in the case of an LPoA, or a doctor, should any of them wish to do so.

So then, what about the circumstance where an elderly patient has no valid Living Will or DNACPR form in place, and does not have the mental capacity to make informed decisions for him/herself? What if they have advanced dementia and/or a lowered level of consciousness, they're deteriorating, and they present with the physiological signs that they're nearing their end of life, what happens then? Do the next-of-kin decide for the patient whether paramedics intervene or not? You would think so, wouldn't you? However, legally, family and friends are not allowed to make that decision for them, unless, that is, they have been appointed as the patient's LPoA. And so to the very similar situation I found myself in during the next particular incident.

It was 3 p.m. on a lovely summer's day. My colleague, Steve, an Emergency Care Assistant, and I were trundling along in the ambulance towards the station, hoping to sit outside and absorb a little sunshine. At 3.15 p.m. the cab radio sounded,

'Go ahead, over.'

'Roger, RED call to Holly Bush Residential Care Home, for a ninety-seven year old female who's deteriorating.'

'Roger, understood, over.'

Steve put his foot down and drove in the direction of the care home. When we arrived on scene, equipment to hand, we were escorted by a member of staff to the patient's ground floor room. The escorting carer then left us with two other members of staff. The patient, Lily, was layed flat on her back on her bed, her eyes closed. My first observation was how frail she looked. She must have been six or seven stone wet through. Her prominent ribs were visible through her nightdress, and her legs weren't much wider than her arms. I could see the rise and fall of her chest at first glance, so I was satisfied that she was breathing, albeit irregularly and a little slower than what is considered 'normal parameters' for an adult; a normal adult respiratory rate is between twelve and twenty breaths per minute.

We'd previously received the information from the ambulance dispatcher that the care staff had called treble-nine because Lily was deteriorating, but I wanted them to elaborate further and so I introduced myself and Steve, and then began questioning one of the care staff in the room.

'What's your main concern today?' I asked.

'Well, Lily hasn't been her usual self over the last two or three days... you know, not as responsive... and she's been refusing food and fluid too,' one carer stated.

'Has her doctor been out to see Lily at all since she's not been her usual self?'

'No, we've not felt the need to call her GP because it's normal for her not to be fully responsive all of the time anyway, but she's worse this afternoon, even less responsive than normal.'

'When you say it's normal for her not to be fully responsive, do you mean she's always asleep or that she has severe dementia, or other condition that causes a lowered level of consciousness?' I asked with relevance.

'Yeah, she has severe dementia, but over the past few weeks she's been generally bedbound and hardly ever awake.'

'I see. Judging by her frailty, I take it she has very little or no mobility then?' I asked.

'That's right, she needs assistance to get out of bed, but she generally doesn't leave this room.'

'Am I right in assuming she has very little quality of life then?' I asked, again with relevance.

'Yeah, she's generally bedbound and is asleep a lot of the time.'

'Can I have a look at her care file please, so I can see her past medical history and current medications?'

'Yeah, I'll go and get it.' The carer left to retrieve Lily's care file, while the other remained in the room, so I began the physical assessment of Lily in order to build a bigger picture of her acute health. I sat on the edge of the bed and took hold of her wrist to palpate for a pulse. It was impalpable. While holding her wrist I noticed that she felt very dry to the touch, and the skin on the back of her hand tented for several seconds when I lightly pinched it; a typical sign of severe dehydration. Then, gazing at her I said,

'Lily, can you hear me?' Her eyes remained closed and no sound emerged from her mouth. 'Lily!' I shouted, as I gently shook her shoulders and pressed on the nail bed of one of her fingers. Again her eyes remained closed, but she did slowly withdraw her hand when I pressed on her nail bed. Based on that response I noted Lily's AVPU as a 'P' – responds to painful stimuli. I then mentally calculated her total GCS as six. She scored one for not opening her eyes to any form of stimuli, one for not responding to my voice, and a four for withdrawing from painful stimuli. I turned to Steve, who was looking on, and said, 'Can you get me a set of obs please, mate, the full hit.' By that I meant everything: sats, respiratory rate, blood pressure, temperature, blood glucose and a 12-lead ECG.

With the patient's implied consent, Steve began obtaining the observations I'd requested. Meanwhile, I began looking through the care file that had by now been retrieved from the office. As I browsed through the file, I made a mental note of Lily's medical history and medications, etcetera. She had chronic kidney disease, which is common in the elderly, and as I'd already learned, severe dementia was documented, amongst many other significant conditions and diseases. She was on an abundance of medications – referred to as polypharmacy – for most of her ailments. I also ascertained that she had no next-of-kin, no LPoA, and there was no ADRT or DNACPR form in place either.

As Steve continued to obtain the observations, the care staff looked on, intermittently providing answers to significant questions that I asked. My questioning centred on ruling in, or out, the potential causes of her presentation, other than the natural causes attributable to old age. After several minutes, Steve's duties now completed, I noted that Lily's sats were ninety-two percent. As already acknowledged on arriving at Lily's side, her respiratory rate was irregular and a little low at between eight and eleven breaths per minute. With those observations jotted down, and on my request, Steve administered oxygen to her while I interpreted the measurements of Lily's other vital signs. Her systolic blood pressure was just 70mmHg. That was low and the reason she had an impalpable pulse in her wrist. Her blood glucose was 5.2mmol/l and her temperature was 36.8 centigrade, both of which were within normal parameters. The most significant finding was her ECG printout. It displayed a heart rate of just 26 BPM. That was profoundly low!

From all of those observations, I was able to build a physiological picture to assist my clinical thought processes. I began to ponder what was the best course of action for Lily, and so I mentally summarised her presenting observations and other information I'd gathered. 'She's ninety-seven years old. She has a GCS of six – therefore, she doesn't have the mental capacity to make decisions for herself.' Though, if she had been fully conscious, severe dementia would highly likely have prevented her from having mental capacity anyway. 'Her sats were ninety-two percent prior to O2 administration. She has a lowered respiratory rate, appears pale, has very low blood pressure, and a very slow heart rate.' That summarised information assisted me to build a clinical picture and make a risk assessment of Lily's acute health status – she was extremely unstable.

What did go through my mind though, based on her presentation, was that Lily was peri-arrest. From many previous experiences where the patient was as unstable as Lily, a simple move from the bed to the stretcher can cause them to take their last breaths and instigate a cardiac arrest. Concerned about that happening, I had to first carefully consider what was in her best interests: Convey her to hospital, with resuscitative measures undertaken from the moment we moved her, or leave Lily at home to die with dignity? However, with no LPoA, no next-of-kin, and no ADRT or DNACPR form in place, I couldn't help but think that I was caught between a rock and a hard place, particularly from an ethical point of view.

The European Court of Human Rights has ruled that: 'Treatment without consent, invasive treatment contrary to a patient's best interest, and withholding medical care' can all be deemed 'inhuman or degrading treatment'. With that in mind, what I had to consider was whether it would be unethical of me to move Lily, instigating a cardiac arrest and to then intervene with resuscitative measures, or whether it would be unethical of me to leave her to die. I turned to face the carers and said,

'Lily is very unstable and death is imminent without invasive treatment. However, my problem is, as Lily doesn't have the mental capacity to make decisions for herself and she has no next-of-kin, no attorney, no Living Will, and no DNACPR in place—'

'There's definitely no DNACPR in place, is there?' Steve said, cutting in on my explanation.

'No, definitely not,' answered the carer. That may seem like a silly question for Steve to have asked, but it wasn't. In the past, prior to this incident, he and I had been dispatched to a Residential Care Home to attend to an elderly patient with dementia, who was in cardiac arrest. We attempted to resuscitate him for almost twenty minutes before a member of the care staff walked into the room and informed us that the patient had a valid DNACPR form in place. She told us that it had been pinned, or blu-tacked, to the wall above the headboard on his bed – the resident had had no idea what the document was. It quickly became apparent that it had fallen off the wall and had landed down the back of his bed. During the previous several days, no member of staff had noticed that the form was no longer on the wall, and they obviously hadn't memorised which residents had a valid DNACPR form in place. Fortunately – although this sounds terrible – resuscitative measures were unsuccessful. I continued to explain to Lily's carers the difficult predicament I was in.

'I'm a little indecisive as to what is the most ethical avenue to take: Withhold treatment and allow her to die here at home, or move her and then attempt to resuscitate her and prolong her life,' I said.

Knowing full well that moving Lily would instigate a cardiac arrest scenario, I stood by the bedside and silently mused a little more. 'Should I gain IV access and administer some atropine? By doing so *may* increase her heart rate and blood pressure high enough to move her without her deteriorating in to cardiac arrest. Then again, atropine might not be effective. What if I do administer atropine and it's effective and so we attempt to move her, but she arrests; do we intervene?'

No health care professional should ever find themselves in the predicament I was in. At the ripe old age of ninety-seven, Lily should have had some legal end of life care plan in place, or at the very least a DNACPR signed by her GP. For some reason – an oversight maybe – I was faced with an ethical dilemma. I pondered some more. 'If I move her I'm going to instigate a cardiac arrest, and chest compressions would obliterate her ribs and potentially puncture her lungs after the first ten. And if that's not bad enough, we'll pump her body with drugs, insert a tube down her windpipe and rush her to hospital, and she will highly likely be confirmed dead and sent to the mortuary with multiple traumatic injuries that she didn't have before *we* arrived! Also, the chance of successful resuscitation is minimal. And if resuscitation is successful, what mental and physical pain would Lily suffer as a consequence of my unethical interventions? She'd never leave hospital! Does she not deserve to have a good death? Should she suffer for longer with no quality of life?'

As far as I was concerned, I'd finally answered my own dilemma just by pondering over the matter. It was a question of ethics. It wouldn't be ethical, morally right or humane to bring such a traumatic and undignified death on this frail old lady in front of me. However, having no legal forms in place, but wanting to leave Lily at home to die in peace, meant I needed a health care professional higher up the hierarchy to strengthen my justification. Somebody who knew Lily better than I did and who would likely agree and deem Lily as nearing her end of life through old age, not by a medical condition that could be treated with such success that it would restore her health to that of several weeks previous. That somebody was Lily's GP.

I contacted him at his surgery and explained the predicament I was in as the attending clinician at *his* patient's bedside. I verbally conveyed Lily's observations and my clinical thought processes, including how I believed moving her would instigate a cardiac arrest, and how traumatic and futile resuscitation would be. I also shared that I strongly believed that leaving Lily to die peacefully at home was acting in her best interests, rather than conveying her to hospital only for the sake of having no ADRT, DNACPR or LPoA in place. Following my explanation, he requested that I remained on scene and he would visit Lily and liaise with me shortly. While waiting for the doctor to arrive, I continued monitoring Lily's vital signs for deterioration, conscious that if she deteriorated considerably before the doctor arrived, I'd have to intervene. Although it would have been against my own ethical intentions of wanting to allow her a dignified death, withholding treatment may have been considered unethical in the eyes of the law, until such time as her doctor confirmed that Lily was nearing her end of life and that no medical intervention would be of any benefit to her quality of life.

I was on tenterhooks for over fifteen minutes, every minute hoping that Lily didn't deteriorate in to cardiac arrest. Fortunately, her GP arrived before Lily's condition worsened. Upon observing her and browsing at my documentation showing her vital signs recorded since arriving at her bedside, he agreed with me, without further question, that she should remain in the care home and that she *was* nearing her end of life; medical intervention and attempting to prolong her life would be unethical and not in her best interest. He signed a DNACPR form and asked the care staff to place Lily on permanent observations and to provide plenty of tender loving care until she passed away peacefully, which we envisaged would be a short time later. He also emphasised that if they had any concerns whatsoever, or if Lily died shortly after him leaving them, then to contact him immediately.

With all ethical decisions agreed, Steve and I vacated the care home and ambled back out to the ambulance, parting from the doctor. A short time later, we cleared with ambulance control and were asked to return to base.

Prior to and since attending to Lily, I've often asked myself, and some of my colleagues, this question: Why is it that health care professionals frequently try to prolong the lives of frail, elderly patients who possess the physiological signs and symptoms of someone naturally nearing their end of life; often a life that has no quality, a mere existence? Or of those who have been collapsed in cardiac arrest for ten or fifteen minutes, when they'd have sustained irreversible brain damage within three to five minutes of them arresting? Is it not a more ethical, humane and morally right choice of care pathway to allow them to die with dignity in their own home, surrounded by their loved ones, or at least by those who care for them and who they're familiar with?

Case in point. A short time after arriving back at the station, a control room dispatcher informed me that a GP had phoned out of courtesy, wanting a message conveyed to the ambulance crew that had attended to one of his patients a short time before. He had just received a phone call from a member of staff at Holly Bush Residential Care Home to report the anticipated death of a resident. It was, of course, Lily. She had died with her carers by her side, naturally and peacefully in her bed, showing no signs of pain or discomfort whatsoever.

The Dark Side

Chapter 10
A Life-Changing Decision

I have attended to countless road traffic collisions involving all forms of transport, including bicycles. Some of those collisions were minor and some of them serious but not immediately life-threatening. Then there were those that left the patient with life-changing disabilities – those patients, though eventually discharged from hospital, were unfortunately left paralysed or severely brain damaged. And then of course there were those that were fatal, either confirmed dead at the scene or confirmed dead at the hospital following a fight to save their life by my colleagues and I, and the A&E doctors and nurses.

Many of the RTCs that I've attended were caused by excess speed, poor negotiation of corners and bends, and/or the driver had been eating, smoking or foolishly using a mobile phone. On some occasions, the collision was caused by the driver being under the influence of drugs and/or alcohol.

It's bizarre, but I've often glanced at a mangled car as I've rolled up at the scene of a collision and very quickly thought, 'That'll be a fatal,' only to find the patient stood by the roadside, red-faced; and not because they were covered in 'claret', just embarrassed by their poor driving standards. Conversely, I've rolled up on scene to find a car with barely any damage, in comparison to other RTCs, only to find the driver or other occupant… dead. I've even known a driver to collide with another car, vacate their vehicle and pace about waiting for the police and ambulance to arrive. Then, witnessed by onlookers, to suddenly collapse onto the tarmac and die! But out of all of the RTCs that I've attended throughout my career so far, the following incident was one of the worst I've had to deal with.

It was 1:25 a.m. on a warm summer's night and I was just over half way through a twelve-hour night shift. My crewmate, Ben, a paramedic, and I had not stopped since we came on duty at 7 p.m., nor had any of the other crews from the same station. We had all been responding to treble-nine after treble-nine and Ben and I were already exhausted, but unfortunately we had over five and half hours of the shift left to go. We were the only crew sat on station, relaxing for the first time that night, when at 1:30 a.m. my hand portable radio sounded.

'Go ahead, over,' I said.

'Roger, RED call to a single vehicle RTC, car versus house, Spa Lane, two female patients reported. Police and fire en route too. I'll send another ambulance when one becomes available, but can you give me a sit-rep on your arrival, over,' the dispatcher said.

'Roger that,' I replied. By 'sit-rep' she meant 'situation report', detailing how many patients there were, how many more ambulances were required, could the fire service be stood down and returned to their station, and so on. So we exited the station and adopted our appointed positions in the ambulance.

While driving towards the location given, which was about six miles from the station, I began to think about the potential injuries each patient might have sustained, bearing in mind that Spa Lane had a sixty miles per hour speed limit. Obviously, that was no guarantee that the motorist had been driving at sixty miles per hour when she collided with the house, but nevertheless I had to prepare for the worst case scenario from what details I knew; anything less would be a bonus, both for all the attending emergency services and the patients themselves. Clearly, crashing into a house at high speed can cause significant, if not fatal injuries.

Physics, particularly Newton's laws of motion, plays a huge part in the thought processes of pre-hospital and in-hospital health care professionals while assessing and treating the occupants of a road traffic collision. For the occupants, the effects of a collision are not complete the moment their vehicle comes to an abrupt halt after hitting a brick wall at potentially sixty miles per hour. Why? Because if unrestrained when the car is suddenly brought to a stop, those inside the vehicle continue to be projected forward at sixty miles per hour. When *they* come to an abrupt halt – and this can be true for those restrained by seat belts, too – their internal organs will still be moving at a rate of 60 MPH. The sheer forces and injuries that can occur throughout that process of physics can cause substantial internal, multi-system trauma.

For example, the head impacting the steering wheel can result in brain trauma, causing brain haemorrhage and potentially brain damage. The impact of the heart against the breastbone can cause the heart to bleed; most likely to be fatal at the scene. The chest impacting the steering wheel can cause a collapsed lung or lungs, and this can progress to what is known as a tension *pneumo*-thorax, or if haemorrhaging of the lungs also occurs, then a tension *haemo-pneumo*-thorax – a bit of a mouthful that one, isn't it! Both can prove fatal if not remedied with the utmost urgency. Other internal organs, such as the liver, kidneys and spleen can tear and be completely severed from their original anatomical positions, as if sliced with a cheese wire. The consequences of any of these impact injuries can include profuse internal bleeding, though sometimes only gradual blood loss occurs and does not initially affect the patient's vital signs. It can be several hours later, when multiple observations have been undertaken in the hospital and x-rays, MRI and CT scans carried out, that internal bleeding is recognised.

If the occupants are restrained and airbags deployed then that *usually* reduces the severity of damage caused by a collision, but cannot completely prevent injury. Although airbags have saved many lives, I've witnessed severe, even fatal injuries despite the intervention of airbags. Most have been noted when the driver's seat was incorrectly positioned and the driver was sat too close to the steering wheel when the collision occurred. When a driver is found slumped over the steering wheel following a collision, it usually means the body or head has absorbed some of the force of the airbag's deployment, rather than the airbag helping to diffuse the force of the collision.

Now that I've explained a little physics, let's move on.

When we arrived at the scene of the collision, Ben parked the ambulance a short distance away, leaving the blue lights flashing and the engine on run-lock. We vacated the cab and donned our high visibility jackets and protective helmets. I grabbed the paramedic and oxygen bag, and also a torch as Spa Lane was a poorly lit, rural stretch of road. Advancing towards the mangled heap of carnage crunched against the house, I noticed several nearby homeowners stood awaiting the emergency services' arrival. None of them were the owners of the house the car had collided with – we quickly learned that they were away on holiday. In some respects, that was a blessing.

While I confirmed the number of patients inside the vehicle and their life-status, Ben briefly liaised with the homeowners. He was informed by one couple that they heard what they described as 'an explosion' while they lay in bed. The noise was in fact the loud bang heard when a car collides with a house at high speed. Judging by the amount of crumple damage visible on my arrival at the vehicle, I estimated the speed of impact to have been approximately fifty miles per hour.

There was utter carnage. The front of the car, including the bonnet, had been severely reduced in size and was covered with rubble. Fortunately, the windscreen didn't have signs of a 'bull's eye'. If it had, that would have suggested that an occupant's head may well have hit the windscreen. There were, however, thousands of cracks in the glass from the impact. Looking at the front side windows, I could only assume that the occupants had been travelling with their windows wound completely down, because there was no evidence of shattered glass on either side.

Due to the damage to the vehicle, I was unable to open the door on either the passenger or driver's side – the energy from the collision had damaged the hinge mechanisms and dented the doors. During the initial outside inspection using the torch, I shone light through the open driver's side window. There, I was presented with a young lady I predicted to be in her early twenties, sat in the passenger seat crying but fully conscious. The driver, however, another young lady in her early twenties, was slumped forward with her head on the steering wheel, her seatbelt still in place and being pulled taut by the weight of her body. She appeared unconscious but, to my relief, she was breathing, albeit slow and deep. A palpable radial and central pulse was also a relief to find.

I was reluctant to climb into the back of the car and assess the patients from the rear seats, so instead leant forward through the driver's side window. It was at that point my olfactory senses smelt strong alcoholic fumes inside the car, potentially being omitted from the breath of the passenger and quite possibly the driver, too! I shone my torch into the back, to ensure there were no other passengers other than the two the dispatcher had mentioned. On further inspection with the torch, it became apparent that there was very little evidence of external bleeding on either of the girls. However, that didn't reduce my concerns, as the state of the car meant severe, life-threatening injuries could be, and probably had been, sustained by both of them. With one patient fully conscious and another unconscious confirmed, I passed my sit-rep to ambulance control, which included a request for a second ambulance when one became available, and to keep the fire service and police responding to the scene. Both patients were trapped inside and potentially bleeding to death internally; we'd therefore need the roof of the car removed as quickly as possible.

Peering in through the window once again, I pointed the torch at the young driver's face. Both of her eyes were closed, but I could hear vague groans coming from her mouth. I noticed that the airbag had been deployed, but obviously by now had fully deflated as it is supposed to within a second of deploying. The airbag being deployed would play a significant part in my thought processes when assessing her vital signs and her injuries, though what initially went through my mind was the fact that she was slumped forward, with her head on the steering wheel, even though her seatbelt was applied.

As mentioned earlier, a patient found slumped forward following a collision usually means that the position of the driving seat is incorrectly adjusted and the driver is sat too close to the steering wheel, so I tried to gauge whether the seat was too close. I believed it was! That concerned me, because it might have been the reason why she was unconscious, and I now began to suspect that she might have a progressing internal head injury; if that were the case, she would need to be transferred to a trauma centre ASAP! Being unconscious was serious enough, but a patient who's unconscious and has a progressing head injury is even worse. I therefore prioritised the unconscious patient and intended to have her removed from the carnage first.

We'd been on scene less than two minutes. Ben was stood on the passenger's side of the vehicle, peering through at the fully conscious, yet understandably upset passenger, trying to calm her and undertake some basic observations on her at the same time. While he was doing that, I leant forward through the driver's side window and began ascertaining some details from the passenger, while also continuing to listen to the groans and sounds of breathing coming from the unconscious driver.

'I know you're scared and upset but try and stay calm and keep still for me. Now, what's your name?'

'Lucy... Is she dead?' she asked, shivering and extremely shaken and upset.

'No, she's not dead, so stay nice and calm, OK. We're gonna help you both, but we're gonna get her out first, though. It's very important that you stay still for now, until another ambulance and the fire service arrive, OK,' I said.

'Is she gonna be alright though, she's not gonna die is she?'

'Just stay calm. Now, what's her name?' I asked.

'Sophie,' she answered.

'OK Lucy, remember what I said, stay still until help arrives. I'm gonna assess and treat Sophie first, alright?' Leaning into the driver's side of the car, I attempted to obtain a response from Sophie using the AVPU scale. 'Sophie! Sophie! Can you hear me?!' I shouted. All I could hear were barely audible groans. With that mentally noted I then applied the sats monitor to her index finger and placed the small, lightweight machine onto her lap and awaited a figure to display.

Given the speed of impact and visible damage present, I would have liked to have immediately immobilised her head and neck, as a c-spine injury was possible. However, once you take hold of the head you're committed and are then unable to do anything else, not even contact ambulance control or undertake any assessments on your patient, because you have no free hands to do either. I didn't want Ben committed to holding Sophie's head for me, or Lucy's head either, because then I'd have lost an assistant, should I have needed his help. Although Sophie was slumped forward on the steering wheel, I daren't pull her back because it needed doing with a little tact in order to minimise the risk of further spinal cord damage, in the event that she'd sustained a spinal cord injury. Therefore, I left the seatbelt in place rather than cut it, because it was keeping her from moving.

Due to her conscious level, the patency of Sophie's airway was at risk. For that reason, I took out a nasopharyngeal airway adjunct from the paramedic bag, applied KY jelly to it and, with the torch in one hand and the airway adjunct in the other, inserted the malleable plastic tube into her right nostril.

Glancing at the sats monitor resting on her lap, I noted the figure; it displayed a sats measurement of ninety-three percent.

'That's a little low, but not too bad,' I thought. With the ambient noise levels reasonably quiet, with the exception of the ambulance engine running nearby, I once again listened to the quality of each of her breaths. Her breathing rate was reduced, so I quickly placed an oxygen mask on the steering wheel so *some* supplemental oxygen would be inhaled without having to move her head to place the mask on her properly.

Stood by the passenger side of the car, Ben continued to question and monitor the upset, traumatised passenger, Lucy. Meanwhile, I continued to monitor Sophie's conscious level, and periodically felt for a pulse in her wrist and neck. I also lifted her right eyelid up and shone my pen torch into her right pupil. The pupil was dilated but did react to the light; granted, a little slower than would normally be expected, but that was a significant sign. Pupils that react to light sluggishly can indicate a progressing head injury. The fact that her pupil was dilated could suggest several things. One, because the ambient light was poor, her pupils would naturally dilate to allow for better night vision. When I shone my pen torch into her eye, it would naturally constrict because it senses the presence of bright light and therefore reacts to reduce the amount of light it allows in.

Another positive sign of Sophie having dilated pupils was that it meant she still had 'sympathetic tone'. What I mean by that is her nervous system still had the capability to speed things up in her body, whereas poor sympathetic tone might have indicated that she had sustained a spinal cord injury. On the other hand, her pupil could also have been dilated because she had consumed alcohol; however, she was in no position to provide a breath test for the police!

I couldn't assess Sophie's left pupil because her head was turned on to her left cheek resting against the steering wheel. To assess her left pupil would have meant moving her, which I didn't want to do until more helping hands had arrived, unless it became absolutely necessary, that is.

Ben and I had only been on scene for several minutes when, fortunately, two fire appliances arrived. I remained where I was, stood next to the driver's side door, monitoring Sophie. The chief of one of the appliances approached me.

'Hiya, what 'ave we got?' he asked.

'Right, there are two females in the front, one fully conscious and another unconscious. I need two of your crew to get in the back and immobilise the head of each of the occupants, and I need the roof off ASAP.'

'Right, OK,' he said.

'How long do you think it'll take, 'cause they've both got the potential for serious injuries but they can't be assessed properly until they're out of the car?'

'We'll 'ave it off in fifteen or twenty minutes,' he said.

'OK, excellent,' I replied.

The fire commander then ordered several of his crew to stabilise the car with cribbing blocks, while two others got inside the car from the rear passenger side doors. After doing so, one reached forward and placed a hand on either side of Sophie's head and, with assistance, carefully moved her backwards so she came to sit upright. Another fireman then applied a rigid collar from the front and secured it in place around Sophie's neck. Once the collar was in place, a further fireman cut the seatbelt, thus freeing Sophie from the restraint. Meanwhile, his colleague took hold of Lucy's head and another applied a rigid collar around her neck, too. It would leave both firemen unavailable to do anything else throughout the entire extrication but, thankfully, there were plenty of them and so I was able to delegate the task to the crew of the fire service.

The rest of the fire crew got to work immediately, and within minutes the visibility became clearer as the fire service scene lights shone down on to the crumpled car. The noise of engines and generators resonated around the crash site. A hydraulic cutter was prepared to enable the roof to be cut off the car, allowing us to work together as a multi-service team to get the young ladies out and into a more suitable position to be assessed and treated. In the background, I could see the reflection of blue flashing lights bouncing off the walls of detached houses; it was the ambulance that I'd requested, approaching the scene, and so I readied myself to delegate the further assessment and treatment of Lucy to them upon liaising with the crew.

When they pulled up on scene, they too donned their protective attire and approached the mangled vehicle. I explained to them the status of both patients and they immediately took over from Ben, who then calmly walked back to our ambulance to fetch all of the immobilisation equipment and the stretcher. There was no rush because both patients were still trapped inside. A short time later, the traffic police arrived. There was little they could do under the circumstances, apart from manage the traffic, which at that time in the morning was minimal.

Meanwhile, the fire crew made the inside of the car safer for both Lucy and Sophie in preparation for when the extrication took place, and also for their own colleagues sat inside immobilising the patients' heads. They used specialised safety equipment called the 'glass management kit' consisting, amongst other items, of a large sheet that covers the occupants and rescuers inside the vehicle, so that when the windscreen is sawn using a reciprocating saw, any shattered glass debris or splinters are prevented from harming anyone inside. They also used protective equipment known as 'tear-drops', made of hard plastic, which they place near the patients' faces while the roof is being cut off. They're called tear-drops because they're moulded in the shape of…well, a tear-drop, of course.

As a fireman began applying the vice-like grip of the hydraulic cutting equipment around the first A-post, Ben returned with all the gear and neatly prepared it, ready for when the roof had been removed and we could commence the careful but swift extrication of the patients. Sophie was my priority and so would be removed first, because her presentation meant she had time-critical features and could therefore deteriorate rapidly, maybe even decline to traumatic cardiac arrest.

The noise around the crash scene was incredible. There were several emergency vehicles on scene, all with their engines running. If that wasn't noisy enough, the use of the fire service's generators and the noise of shattering glass and metal being cut made it even noisier. In fact it was so loud that whenever anybody spoke they had to shout at the top of their voices.

Within fifteen minutes, the 'A', 'B' and 'C' posts had been cut. Four firemen stepped forward and took a corner each and raised the roof, with windscreen attached, completely separating it from the rest of the car, before walking backwards in a synchronised manner and placing it onto the ground. Working with the fire service as a multi-disciplined team, we proceeded to prepare Sophie to be removed from the vehicle using the longboard. The plan was to maintain the immobilisation of her head and roll the backrest of Sophie's seat as far as it would go. We would then carefully slide the longboard down between her back and the backrest, as far down to her backside as possible. Once positioned, we would use a synchronised method where only one person is in command. The person taking lead would be charged with giving instructions to slide Sophie gradually up the board until she lay completely flat.

So with the roof removed, we worked to implement that plan. After five or six minutes of meticulous negotiation of the longboard, Sophie was finally in situ on the stretcher. It was only after Sophie had been removed from the car that her accurate GCS became clear to me. Looking at her lying flat, I noticed her arms were flexing towards her chest, as if trying to catch a ball. That wasn't a voluntary action by Sophie; it was the involuntary action called 'decorticate posturing'. Decorticate posturing is a sign that there is damage to the nerve pathway between the brain and spinal cord, so I quickly made a mental calculation of Sophie's GCS. It was six. She scored a one for not opening her eyes throughout my entire time on scene so far with her; a two for making incomprehensible sounds only; and a three for having decorticate posturing. A GCS of six was dire and, unbeknown to me at the time, the prognosis would begin to look bleaker as time went on.

While Ben placed the oxygen mask now fully over Sophie's face, I once again assessed her pupillary reaction to light, only this time I was able to assess both of her eyes. Sophie's pupils still reacted sluggishly to my pen-torch light but remained equal and dilated. Therefore, it came as a relief that there was no evidence of a blown pupil. What I mean by that is when a light is shone into the eyes, one pupil remains permanently fixed and dilated and, therefore, appears larger than the other pupil. This is often the case when someone sustains a significant head injury from, for instance, impacting the steering wheel or windscreen. Usually within minutes, the internal bleeding inside the closed box – that is, the skull – can cause pressure to build up, causing the oculomotor nerve to become compressed. The oculomotor nerve is the third of twelve paired cranial nerves in the brain and controls most of the eye's movements, including constriction of the pupil. When the oculomotor nerve is compressed, or damaged by a lesion in the nerve, it can cause a pupil to blow.

Another side effect of a head injury is cerebral irritation. This causes the patient, through no fault of their own, to involuntarily thrash about and, if conscious, often hurl obscenities at the ambulance crew or anyone else around them trying to help. It has to be said that when you witness this, it is quite disturbing because the prognosis is poor. Unless the pressure is released – by those fantastic neurosurgeons who drill into the skull – the pressure increases and pushes the brain down through the small opening at the base of the skull; a term called 'coning'. Once coning occurs, the patient is likely to die… or remain on a ventilator, keeping the patient alive until the decision is made by the family to switch the machine off. In the event the patient regains consciousness, there's a chance that they'll be severely brain damaged and live – if you can call it that – in a vegetative state for the rest of their life.

Ben and I began the process of applying the straps across Sophie's chest and legs, and a figure-of-eight around her lower legs and feet. We were almost complete; all I had to do before finishing off the immobilisation process was to check the orifices of her ears to look for CSF fluid, a clear, colourless bodily fluid found in the brain and spine. Some patients who sustain a significant head injury leak CSF fluid from their ears. On close inspection, Sophie's ears were not leaking any fluid at all. With that confirmed, we finished off the immobilisation process by applying head blocks to either side of her head, before securing them in place with a Velcro strap across her forehead and under the chin section of the rigid neck collar. Then we carefully wheeled her into the saloon of the ambulance.

After securing the stretcher in place, it was time to fully assess Sophie before conveying a pre-alert message to ambulance control. Time was of the essence if Sophie had sustained a head injury, and so Ben and I worked in a measured but hurried manner. Stood in the back of the ambulance, I turned to Ben and said, with a sense of urgency in my voice,

'Right, listen up mate. Get me a BP, blood glucose, and get the three lead ECG on her as quick as you can, while I get IV access.' While Ben carried out his designated tasks, I rummaged through the cupboard drawer for the cannulation equipment. Then, I applied a tourniquet to Sophie's right arm and patted her hand where the vein was engorging with blood. Due to decorticate posturing, I had to extend her arm in order to cannulate, and that proved difficult as the flexing was an involuntary action. Nevertheless, with perseverance I managed to obtain IV access.

Within minutes, Ben had undertaken the observations I'd asked him to. I glanced at the ECG monitor displaying her heart rate of 125 BPM. Her systolic blood pressure measured 123mmHg. I began pondering for a moment while looking at the figures displayed on the monitor, and then it dawned on me: 'She's got internal bleeding somewhere other than her head!' I thought.

Based on the decorticate posturing displayed by her flexed arms, I believed Sophie had sustained a significant head injury. Normally, a patient with such an injury would possess a high systolic blood pressure. Sophie's blood pressure wasn't that high. That caused unease, because a normal or low blood pressure in conjunction with a head injury could suggest there's significant internal or external bleeding present. Given the position of the car seat Sophie had been sat in, I could only assume she had fractured her pelvis and possibly fractured her femur, or even both of her femurs, although there were no obvious signs of fractured femurs while she lay on the stretcher – no obvious deformity, anyway. While deformity is not always present, it's often quite easy to spot fractured femurs, whether your patient is clothed or not.

I hadn't got to the point of cutting her clothes off ready for the A&E consultant to undertake both his primary and secondary survey upon our arrival at A&E. Nevertheless, I had to treat my suspicions. So directing my gaze at Ben, I said,

'Set me up a fluid as quick as you can mate, I wanna get going in a minute.'

'Yep, will do,' he replied.

A minute or so later, Ben handed me the prepared bag of fluid, so I hung it up and attached the giving set to the cannula in Sophie's arm, and opened the clamp just enough to allow a small amount to drip slowly through her veins. Once I was satisfied the fluid was dripping and that Sophie's flexed arms weren't obstructing it from flowing, I progressed to the next stage of my assessment. I took hold of my tuffcut scissors and started cutting Sophie's top off, from the bottom upwards, carefully skirting under the immobilisation straps. Leaving her bra in place for the purposes of pre-hospital dignity, I then proceeded to remove her shoes and also cut off the rest of her clothes, with the exception of her underwear, from the bottom of her jeans upwards, in order to expose her whole body. I then covered her with several blankets to keep her warm, and also to maintain her dignity and modesty when we removed her from the ambulance upon arriving at the A&E department. Now that Sophie had been appropriately assessed, treated and packaged, so to speak, we were ready to convey her under emergency driving conditions to the hospital.

'Right, Ben, get on to ambulance control and tell 'em to alert A 'n' E. I want a full trauma team including anaesthetist. Tell them RTC, car versus house at approximately one-twenty a.m. Female driver, early twenties, GCS six, query closed head injury, abnormal flexion of the arms. And give them her other obs too. Then get us in quick, mate!'

'OK mate,' Ben replied.

While monitoring Sophie en route and undertaking further blood pressure measurements, along with additional tests, I noticed that Sophie's arms had altered from the flexed position to the extended position, a condition known as 'decerebrate posturing', which suggested that by now she could be coning. The fact that her arms had now become extended, from their previous flexed position, meant that her GCS score had lowered by one. Consequently, her GCS was now five out of a possible fifteen. The prognosis was looking bleak and I wasn't anticipating any kind of happy ending to this traumatic incident.

When we arrived at A&E, Ben parked up in the ambulance bay,

vacated his seat and quickly opened the rear doors, lowering the ramp. We wheeled the stretcher inside and swiftly lifted the longboard onto the resuscitation bed. The room was by now swarming with medical staff. Stood as composed as I could be under the circumstances, I began my handover to the lead doctor.

'This is Sophie. I estimate she's in her early twenties. Sophie is the driver of a car that collided into a house at approximately fifty miles per hour at about one-twenty a.m. Seatbelt worn, airbag deployed but her seat was too close to the steering wheel in my opinion.

'On arrival, Sophie was slumped forward with her head on the steering wheel, being held taut by the seatbelt.

'Airway patent but nasal airway inserted and tolerated. O2 administered.

'On examination, breathing rate slow and deep. She has had palpable radial and carotid pulses throughout. BP one hundred and twenty-three systolic, and her heart rate was one hundred and twenty-five BPM. Blood glucose five.

'Following extrication I noticed abnormal flexion of the arms, which progressed to abnormal extension en route. Query significant closed head injury.

'Her pupils are currently equal and dilated but react sluggishly to light. Mechanism of injury cannot rule out spinal, femur or pelvic injury.

'Patient's clothes cut off post immobilisation, but no secondary survey carried out. Large bore IV cannula inserted into her right arm and a bag of fluid hung up on a slow drip.

'Are there any questions?'

'No, thank you... well done,' the doctor replied, looking alternately between me and Sophie.

Within a few minutes of arriving at A&E, Sophie had been anaesthetised, intubated and attached to a ventilator. She was also catheterised, and had another large bore cannula inserted into her left arm and blood samples taken from within.

Lucy arrived at hospital by ambulance a short time after us, as too did the attending traffic police. Lucy was immediately assessed and stabilised, and although her condition wasn't as serious as Sophie's, she had sustained a fractured pelvis. As Lucy was conscious throughout, the police had been able to ascertain a history of events leading up to the crash. It emerged that Sophie and Lucy had been to a nightclub, and while Sophie had not intended to drink, she had done, but instead of taking a taxi home or arranging for someone to pick her up, she had made the decision to drive while under the influence of alcohol.

During our time in the A&E department completing paperwork, cleaning the inside of the ambulance, replacing stock and grabbing a cup of tea, Sophie received a CT scan and x-rays. The CT scan confirmed a significant head injury. The x-ray confirmed a closed fractured femur and a fractured pelvis, which is why her blood pressure wasn't consistent with a head injury. The bleeding inside her pelvis was a physiological compensatory mechanism that caused her blood pressure to remain quite normal for her age throughout the incident, and therefore mask the typical high blood pressure associated with a closed head injury.

While I was still in the A&E department, Sophie's parents

arrived and were escorted to the resus cubicle, and as you can imagine they were devastated to see their daughter lying on a bed with a tube down her throat and wired up to several machines, and with an abundance of doctors surrounding her. It wasn't a nice experience to witness, because the doctors had to be upfront and honest with them. Sophie's parents were informed that her injuries were life-threatening and that she might not survive through the night. It would be determined by how severe the head injury was and how quickly she received emergency neurosurgery.

Several months went by and I'd heard no more about Sophie since the night I'd attended to her, other than reading about her in the local rag and that she had survived the accident following surgery. Then, while in the corridor of the hospital and passing a nurse I knew and who was still involved in the on-going rehabilitation and care of Sophie, I was able to find out what had happened to her in the short time after the crash, and also ask how Sophie had done to that day. The nurse confirmed that Sophie had received emergency surgery, which I already knew from what I'd read in the newspaper, but went on to tell me that Sophie had been admitted to the Intensive Treatment Unit (ITU) and, following progressive recovery, was then moved into another ward. However, as a result of her injuries, she initially lost all of her independence and was confined to her hospital bed, only moving from there with assistance. She was only partially sighted, and also suffered from frequent seizures. And although she was able to vaguely recognise the voices of her immediate family, she had difficulty speaking and was therefore unable to communicate with them.

A further few months later, while stood outside of the A&E

department, I had to do a double-take when Sophie walked passed me. Yes, walked passed me! She was independently strolling along with her physiotherapist, chatting. The physio was pushing a wheelchair, I assume in case Sophie became too tired to walk. Understandably, Sophie didn't recognise me, as she wouldn't have had any recollection of what followed after she'd crashed her car on that fateful, warm summer's night. What troubled me, though, was how different she looked. She'd lost quite a lot of weight and so appeared petite and almost child-like. Nevertheless, she was up on her feet and making positive progress. Considering the injuries she sustained on that eventful night, I hadn't expected her to be alive several months later, let alone walking along the hospital grounds.

It was a couple of months after that, as I once again passed the nurse who had cared for Sophie, that I learned she had not only been discharged but had the majority of her eyesight back too, and was now able to communicate with her family. However, on asking the nurse whether Sophie would be able to return to her job as a hair stylist, she said,

'No, sadly not.'

Unfortunately, Sophie's attention span was too short and she would therefore not be able to concentrate for long enough to carry out any sort of work. She was also too scared to be on her own, too scared to leave the house, even with her family, and too scared to get into a car, even if it would be driven by one of her own parents. Furthermore, she had recurrent cold sweats, nightmares, anxiety attacks and was diagnosed with post-traumatic epilepsy, and had been prescribed drugs as a consequence. Sophie may have to live with those fears, and the side effects of her traumatic experience, for the rest of her life;

all as a result of that life-changing decision to drive while under the influence of alcohol.

Epilogue

Well there you have it, another selection of my Real Life Accounts. I do hope you've enjoyed reading *The Dark Side Part 2* as much as I enjoyed writing it, and hopefully it has given you a realistic flavour of how unpredictable each shift can be for paramedics, and provided a true insight into the risk assessments and thought processes considered throughout each patient encounter; not forgetting the various emotions we frequently experience, too. Of course, there are more memories I could share with you, some in great detail and others… well, only brief memories have remained. For example, the door supervisor who was shot in the neck at point-blank range by a hooded youth ejected from the public house for refusing to remove the hood from his head. The bullet tore straight through the family man's spinal cord, consequently leaving him paralysed from the neck down.

Then there's the elderly man, a retired Special Police Constable, who, one Halloween night, gave chase to several youths after he caught them throwing eggs at his kitchen window. He collapsed and died of a heart attack in front of his wife.

As tragic as the above examples are, along with some of those accounts you read earlier, I wouldn't want to finish this book by leaving you with the perception that it's all 'dark' and there isn't a *'Lighter Side'* to the profession. Ambulance personnel are very often party to humorous and circumstantial incidents too. Take the following examples as just two of many that I could share with you.

My friend, Geoff, and his crewmate attended to an elderly lady who, following assessment, needed admitting to hospital.

They'd assisted her onto the carry-chair in order to lift her down a flight of stairs. Geoff held the top end of the chair while his crewmate held the bottom end. Now, there was a time when NHS Ambulance Service uniform shirts had Velcro across the top pockets, and you could have your name and job title embroidered into a cloth badge with the corresponding Velcro on the back of it.

At the time of this incident, Geoff's pocket had a strip of Velcro sewn onto it, but he'd forgotten to attach his name badge on to his clean shirt. While lifting the old lady down the stairs, with her sat upright, part of her wig became stuck to the Velcro strip. As they slowly and carefully stepped down each stair, the old lady's wig began to ease gradually backwards off her head and on to Geoff's shirt pocket!

The confused old lady was completely unaware of what was happening to her wig as they were descending the stairs. Unable to stop and let go of the chair mid-way down, Geoff had no choice but to let the wig be pulled further and further from the old lady's head with each step, while chuckling to himself and fighting to keep a strong grip of the carry-chair. By the time they got to the bottom of the stairs, the wig was entirely attached to Geoff's pocket, and all he could see was the now almost bald head of the old lady.

Unable to contain themselves, Geoff and his crewmate had to finally laugh out loud then compose themselves and explain to the old lady that her wig had fallen off, respectfully asking her if she would care to put it back into its correct position.

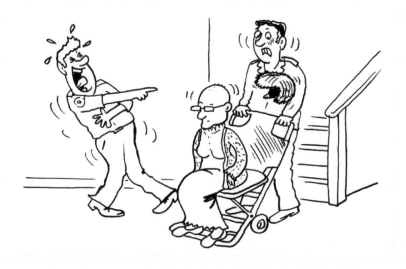

My second example is when my crewmate, Adam, and I were dispatched to attend to an elderly male patient reportedly having a stroke. On arriving inside the bungalow, I eagerly asked the treble-nine caller, the patient's wife, where her husband was. Very calmly, she informed me that he was in the bathroom. So Adam and I rushed to the bathroom situated along the hallway.

The bathroom door was closed and so, anticipating that the patient might be slumped on the other side, I slowly and carefully opened it, not wanting the door to bang against him. As I opened the door, peeking my head around it, I was shocked to find the gentleman with his face covered in shaving foam... stood having a shave!

'What the hell...?' I thought, 'That's not the typical presentation of someone having a stroke!' Baffled, I asked him to go into the lounge to have a chat as to the reasons why we were there. So, sat in the lounge with the patient and his wife, I began ascertaining some information.

'So, what's the concern here this morning?' I asked the lady.

'Well, he woke up this morning a little confused and he can't remember things from yesterday. And he was talking a bit gobbledygook, if you know what I mean?'

'Mmm,' I responded with a nod. 'And in your opinion is he back to normal now?'

'Yes, sort of.'

'OK, good.'

Adam and I then undertook some thorough further questioning and observations. While doing so, his wife informed us that they were supposed to be going to Buckinghamshire that day – which was over one hundred miles away from their address – to visit their son, but had now decided against it. She chose to telephone her son in our presence to let him know, and that telephone conversation went something like this:

'Hiya, love, I've got the paramedics here at the moment. Your dad took a funny turn this morning.' She paused while her son spoke and then said, 'Yeah, we're not gonna come now Son, not while he's been funny.' A brief pause came again. Then she said, 'I don't know what they're gonna do with him yet, they've not said because they're still doing tests on him.' At that point, while Adam and I were crouched alongside each other continuing to assess the patient, I whispered to her,

'Do you want me to talk to him and explain things clearer?'

'Hang on Son, the paramedic's saying something,' she said, before covering the telephone receiver with her hand. 'What did you say, my love?' she asked me.

'I said do you want me to talk to him and explain things

clearer?'

'You can't, love, he's miles away, in Buckinghamshire,' she replied, before carrying on talking to her son. Adam and I just looked at each other, our jaws on the floor, bamboozled by her reply.

'Did I just hear right then, that I can't speak to him because he's in Buckinghamshire? What the hell difference does that make, he's on the telephone?!' I whispered to Adam, with a huge grin on my face.

She never did pass me the telephone to speak to her son, and so I didn't get the chance to explain to him what my clinical impression of his dad was. Every so often throughout the rest of the shift, Adam and I would chuckle to ourselves recalling the sweet old lady's illogical comment.

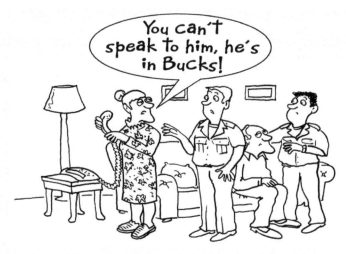

So, with the above humorous anecdotes in mind, the next time you see or hear an ambulance responding to an emergency, don't necessarily assume that the crew is responding to a patient who's experiencing agonising chest or abdominal pain, for example, or sustained serious, life-changing injuries following an RTC, or someone only minutes from death. You never know, it might just turn out to be one of those incidents that causes laugh out loud moments destined to be recited in various mess rooms of various ambulance stations. It might even find its way in to a book.

If, however, *you* are unfortunate enough to find yourself requiring an emergency ambulance, then please rest assured that the crew that arrives at your side is highly likely to be one or more very caring, compassionate health care professionals who wish to deliver the highest standard of patient care. We may be a *Jack of All Trades, Master of None*, but it's the abundance of skills we learn as paramedics that equips us to cope when faced with situations so diverse, demanding and often very sad that even friends, family and some of my patients tell me my job is a thankless one. I'm always compelled to disagree. I am often thanked personally by patients or their loved ones, but saving a life, helping to bring another new life into the world, or just seeing a smile after giving a little TLC, that's all the thanks we need.

Layman's Terms

A Jolly: A holiday or time out from the confines of prison.

A&E: Accident & Emergency.

ABC: Airway, Breathing and Circulation.

Adrenaline: A drug used in cardiac arrest and other medical emergencies to increase blood pressure and cardiac output.

ADRT: Advanced Decision to Refuse Treatment – a Living Will.

Ambulance Dispatcher: A senior Ambulance Service control room operator who dispatches the nearest health care professional/s to the location or address of a patient.

Ambulance Technician: A lesser qualified and skilled member of an ambulance crew.

Analgesic: Pain relief.

Anaphylactic Shock: A potentially life-threatening allergic reaction that can develop rapidly.

Aspirin: An antiplatelet, anti-pyrexic and analgesic drug.

Asystole: A 'flatline' ECG rhythm – signifying the heart is no longer pumping blood and there is no electrical cardiac activity occurring.

Atropine: A drug used to increase the heart rate.

AVPU Scale: A method of assessing a patient's level of consciousness by determining whether a patient is Alert, responsive to Verbal or Painful stimuli, or Unresponsive. Used principally in the initial assessment.

205

BVM: Bag Valve Mask – used to ventilate patients who are not breathing, or are breathing inadequately.

Cannula: A needle for inserting into a vein to administer drugs and/or fluids.

Cannulation: The skill of inserting a needle into a vein, then withdrawing the needle, leaving a plastic tube in place, to administer drugs and/or fluids.

Cardiac Arrest: An absence of breathing and a pulse.

Carotid Pulse: A pulse point located in the neck. Usually signifies a systolic blood pressure of at least 60mmHg.

Claret: Blood.

Control Room Call-Taker: A control room operator who ascertains information from a caller when they telephone the UK ambulance service via a 999 or a 111 call.

CPR: Cardio-Pulmonary Resuscitation – the process of attempting to resuscitate someone by mechanically emulating the work of the heart and lungs by compressing the chest and blowing air into the lungs.

C-spine: The cervical spine – housed and protected by the first seven vertebrae in the spinal column.

Defibrillator: A machine which delivers controlled electric energy across the chest to make the heart restart when it has stopped beating effectively.

Diastolic: The arterial pressure during the relaxing phase of the heart.

Diazemuls: An anti-convulsant/muscle relaxing drug.

DNACPR: Do Not Attempt Cardiopulmonary Resuscitation.

ECA: Emergency Care Assistant.

Entonox: Gas and air – an analgesic.

Epi-pen: An adrenaline auto-injector, used by people with a known or unknown allergy, to deliver a prescribed dose of adrenaline as and when required.

ETA: Estimated Time of Arrival.

Femur: Thigh bone.

GCS: Glasgow Coma Scale/Score – a neurological scale that aims to give a reliable, objective way of recording the conscious state of a person for initial as well as subsequent assessments. A patient is assessed against the criteria of the scale, and the resulting points give a patient a score between 3, indicating deep unconsciousness or an absence of breathing and a pulse, and 15, alert and responsive.

Giving Set: Fluid administration equipment.

GTN: A vasodilation drug used to treat heart conditions, such as heart attacks, angina and chronic heart failure.

Haemorrhaging: Bleeding.

Handover: To verbally convey information about a patient, from one health care professional to another.

HCM: Hypertrophic Cardiomyopathy is a disease affecting the heart muscle.

Heparin: A blood thinner.

HMP: Her Majesty's Prison.

Hydrocortisone: Hydrocortisone is in a class of drugs called steroids. It prevents the release of substances in the body that cause inflammation.

Hypertension: High blood pressure.

Hyperventilating: Rapid, shallow breathing.

Hypovolaemic Shock: Shock due to insufficient blood volume, either from haemorrhage or other loss of fluid, or from widespread vasodilation, so that the blood volume present cannot maintain normal tissue perfusion.

Hypoxia: Inadequate oxygen in the tissues of the body.

Immobilisation: A process of limiting movement, or making incapable of movement.

Inmate: A prisoner.

Intubation: The skill of placing a tube down a patient's windpipe in order to ventilate them when they're not breathing, or breathing inadequately.

IV Glucose: A bag of fluid containing 10% glucose, used to treat hypoglycaemic patients.

Laceration: A cut of any size.

Laryngoscope: A handle with a rigid, blunt, curved blade equipped with a source of light, used for moving a patient's tongue to the left to view the vocal chords.

Longboard: Rigid, stretcher-like equipment used for immobilising and securing suspected spinal cord injured patients prior to their removal from the scene.

LPoA: Lasting Power of Attorney.

Mess Room: A social/refreshment lounge within the ambulance station.

Metoclopramide: An anti-nausea/anti-sickness drug.

Minger: An unpleasant, unhygienic or smelly person.

Morphine Sulphate: An opiate-based analgesic.

NEB: Nebuliser – used to administer Salbutamol and some other drugs in vapour form.

NPA: Nasopharyngeal airway – a small tube inserted into a nostril to provide a patent airway.

'O' Negative Blood: The universal blood group that can be infused into anyone regardless of their specific blood group type.

Paramedic Bag: A bag/rucksack containing the majority of equipment a paramedic will ever need, excluding the bulky equipment.

Peri-arrest: Peri-arrest is a medical term used to describe a patient who is potentially only minutes from cardiac arrest.

Piriton: An anti-histamine drug.

Pre-alert: A message conveyed to a hospital department prior to the arrival of the patient by ambulance.

PRF: Patient Report Form.

Prison Hooch: An alcoholic drink manufactured by inmates.

PTS: Patient Transport Service – the non-emergency aspect of the NHS Ambulance Service.

Pyrexic: A high temperature.

Radial Pulse: A pulse point located in the wrist. Usually signifies a systolic blood pressure of at least 80mmHg.

Rectal: Back passage.

RED Call: 999 Emergency requiring visual and audible warning devices to be utilised while en route to the location of a patient.

Respiratory Arrest: A patient who has ceased breathing, but still has a pulse.

Resus: Resuscitation department – for severely sick or injured patients.

Rigid C-spine Collar: A device used to immobilise a patient's neck or c-spine.

Rigor Mortis: Post death stiffening of the body.

RRV: Rapid Response Vehicle – manned by a solo responder, usually a paramedic, but technicians do man them in some ambulance services.

RTC: Road Traffic Collision.

Salbutamol: A drug that relaxes muscles in the airways and increases air flow to the lungs.

Sats/SP02: A measure of how oxygenated the blood is.

Scoop: A stretcher that divides in two halves – used for lifting patients from the ground onto an ambulance stretcher.

Scran: Slang for food. 'Neck a bit of scran' – to grab something to eat.

Scrote: A male with low character, who is idle, thoughtless, inconsiderate, disrespectful, with bad manners, no moral fibre and often with a poor appearance.

Silent MI: A heart attack where the victim does not experience chest pain.

Situation Report: A report giving the situation of an incident, from an attending crew's perspective – also called a SIT-REP.

SoCO: Scenes of Crime Officers.

Sodium Chloride: 0.9% saline fluid – used to flush cannulas or increase the body's internal fluid volume.

Sphygmomanometer: Equipment for measuring blood pressure.

Status Epilepticus: A continuous seizure lasting for at least 20-30 minutes, or two or more discrete seizures between which the patient does not regain consciousness.

Stethoscope: An acoustic medical device for listening to internal sounds in a human.

Suction Device: A device used to clear blood, saliva, vomit or other secretions from the airway.

Systolic: The arterial pressure during contraction of the heart.

Tenecteplase: A clot-busting drug.

Thrombolysis: A procedure where a clot busting drug is administered IV.

Tourniquet: A constricting device used to allow blood to engorge the veins prior to cannulating.

Trauma Team: A group of doctors and nurses on standby to receive a trauma patient from an ambulance crew.

Triage: A French word meaning 'to sort'. Patients are triaged to enable an order of priority for assessment and treatment from health care professionals.

Tuffcut Scissors: Robust scissors used in emergency medical response and rescue to cut through clothing – for example, leather motorcycle jackets, trousers, boots etc.

12-Lead ECG: Only 10 leads to be precise, but it analyses the rhythm of the heart from 12 different angles. Used to assist a paramedic diagnose various conditions. However, its primary purpose is to diagnose heart attacks.

Ventilating: Assisting a patient to breathe using manual or mechanical means.

Vital Signs (Vitals): The key signs that are used to evaluate the patient's overall condition, including respiratory rate, pulse, blood pressure, level of consciousness, skin characteristics and much more.

Lightning Source UK Ltd.
Milton Keynes UK
UKHW021929140319
339169UK00012B/186/P